List of Contributors

JO ANNE BOORKMAN
Carlson Health Sciences Library
University of California, Davis
Davis, CA

PAMELA BROADLEY
Dartmouth College
Hanover, NH

JAMES A. CURTIS
Health Sciences Library
University of North Carolina
Chapel Hill, NC

DIANE L. FISHMAN
Health Sciences Library
University of Maryland
Baltimore, MD

DIANE FOXMAN FUTRELLE
Medical Center Library
Duke University
Durham, NC

JUDITH M. JOHNSON
The Healthcare Forum
San Francisco, CA

JUDITH A. OVERMIER
School of Library and Informa-
tion Studies
The University of Oklahoma
Norman, OK

TAYLOR PUTNEY
Mead Data Central
Dayton, OH

FRED W. ROPER
University of South Carolina
Columbia, SC

FRIEDA WEISE
Health Sciences Library
University of Maryland
Baltimore, MD

Introduction to Reference Sources in the Health Sciences

FRED W. ROPER

and

JO ANNE BOORKMAN

Third Edition

Medical Library Association
and
The Scarecrow Press, Inc.
Metuchen, N.J., & London
1994

British Library Cataloguing-in-Publication data available

Library of Congress Cataloging-in-Publication Data

Introduction to reference sources in the health sciences / [compiled]
  by Fred W. Roper and Jo Anne Boorkman. — 3rd ed.
     p. cm.
  Includes bibliographical references and index.
  ISBN 0-8108-2889-8 (acid-free paper)
    1. Reference books—Medicine—Bibliography. 2. Medicine—Bibliography.
  3. Medicine—Information services.   I. Roper, Fred W. (Fred Wilburn)
  II. Boorkman, Jo Anne.
  Z6658.I54   1994
  [R118.6]
  610'.72—dc20   94-10708

To
Madonna Stoehr
whose industriousness,
ingenuity, and attention to
detail considerably facilitated
the completion of the manuscript.

CONTENTS

PREFACE

The reception of the first two editions of *Introduction to Reference Sources in the Health Sciences* has been most gratifying. Our intention was to begin work on a third edition immediately after publication of the second edition, to keep the publication up-to-date both for the library school student and for the practicing librarian. It is hard to believe that almost ten years have passed since the publication of the second edition. Needless to say, there have been many changes in reference publications in the health sciences, most notably the emergence of many sources in a variety of electronic formats. Our purpose remains the same—to discuss various types of reference and information sources and their use in reference work in the health sciences, regardless of format.

We have again been selective, choosing those tools that librarians may use on a daily basis in reference work in the health sciences—those tools that may be considered foundation or basic works. Some of the major specialized tools have been included, but there is no attempt to go into subject specialization in great detail. Emphasis is placed on U. S. publications and libraries, although an attempt has been made to address Canadian publications and needs.

The major portions of the book again present the different types of bibliographic and informational sources. Each chapter contains a discussion of the general characteristics of the type of source being considered, followed by examples of the most important tools in the area. In this edition the chapter on Health Legislation Sources has been dropped. Chapter 5 has been renamed Electronic Bibliographic Databases to reflect the changes in these sources and Chapter 11 has been expanded as Audiovisual, Microcomputer and Multimedia Reference Sources. Emphasis is on the use of materials, and, where available, a comparison with similar materials is included. If available, readings are again included for each topic.

Since no consensus exists as to what constitutes "basic works," the materials represent the authors' candidates for such a list. In many instances, other equally appropriate examples could have been selected. For certain groups of sources, e.g., technical report literature, materials that are considerably broader in scope than the health sciences field alone have been included to help the reader toward a clear understanding of the use of these sources in reference work in the health sciences.

Many people have played important roles in the production of this third edition. The chapter authors were prompt and responsive to the deadlines that we faced. Their chapters show their expertise, experience, and enthusiasm for their respective topics. Three chapters from the second edition have been revised by new authors. These authors are indebted to Julie Kuenzel Kwan, J. Michael Homan, and Pamela Broadley for the excellent groundwork that they laid for this edition in preparing the chapters in the second edition. We would be remiss if we did not acknowledge their contributions to this edition. Thanks go to Tom Fleming for providing information on some Canadian sources otherwise unavailable to the authors. The survey of academic and hospital reference services was partially funded by the University of California Research Grants for Librarians Program, Davis Division.

Linda Williams deserves thanks for her work indexing the third edition. Special thanks go to Gayle Sykes and Madonna Stoehr at the College of Library and Information Science, University of South Carolina for their assistance with final manuscript preparation.

Fred W. Roper
Jo Anne Boorkman
November 1993

PART I

The Reference Collection

CHAPTER 1

Organization and Management of the Reference Collection

Jo Anne Boorkman

INTRODUCTION

This book introduces a number of works considered to be desirable tools in a health sciences library's reference collection. All are appropriate, if not essential, for a large library. Smaller libraries will need to be selective in acquiring the most appropriate tools for their collections. First, however, it seems appropriate to explore the nature of the reference collection: how it differs from other parts of the library's collection, what characterizes the materials in it, and how these are selected, organized, and maintained.

Reference collections evolve and develop from the nature of reference work. In addition to carrying out literature searches, reference librarians are most frequently called on for assistance in answering factual and bibliographic questions. The tools most frequently used to answer these types of questions make up the reference collection; materials in this collection are consulted for specific and immediate information instead of being read from beginning to end. To assure that these materials are available for immediate and short-term use, the reference collection is separated from the circulating collections of the library, placed in an easily accessible library service area, and made noncirculating. It should be noted that some medical reference tools require the assistance of a trained librarian for effective use. As reference tools are acquired in electronic format, this assistance takes on additional importance, since the librarian becomes involved with instruction in effective use of the equipment as well as the reference material.

Little has been written on the nature of the reference collection and of the policies for developing and maintaining it [1]. A written collection development policy is a very useful tool and, like other library policies, has a variety of uses. In a time of limited resources, it helps define the scope of the collection for greater selection consistency and wiser use of resources. It can be used to train new staff and help orient them to the nature of reference work in a particular library. It can be used for evaluation of current and future needs based on user queries, new curriculum and research demands, and new technological developments. It can also be useful in defining areas of cooperative collection building with neighboring libraries, or in large academic institutions, with other campus libraries.

Selection policies [2-4], while generally discussing the collection as a whole, usually define four levels of coverage for subject areas: exhaustive/comprehensive, research, reference, and skeletal. These can be described as follows.

1. *Exhaustive.* For a subject collected on the exhaustive level, the library will obtain copies of all editions of all books, journals, pamphlets, reports, and so on, dealing with the subject and published at any time in any language. All manuscript materials relating to this subject will also be acquired.
2. *Research.* For a subject collected on the research level, the library will obtain a current or best edition of the books, journals, pamphlets, reports, and documents in the commonly used languages that are necessary to permit independent research on a doctoral level.
3. *Reference.* For a subject collected on the reference level, the library will obtain a current dictionary, a current encyclopedia, the latest or best editions of several texts, a comprehensive bibliography, one or more journals, an indexing or abstracting journal, and one or more histories.
4. *Skeletal.* For a subject collected on the skeletal level, the library will obtain a current dictionary, the latest or best edition of one or two texts, and a history [5].

Regardless of the level at which the material is collected, the subject should be represented in both the reference and general collections of the library. Therefore, simply defining a level of coverage does not adequately answer the question, "Which materials should comprise a reference collection?"

A reference collection policy should be developed as a document parallel to the overall collection development policy of the library. It should be defined not only in relation to the research and educational goals of the particular institution but also in relation to the types of materials most often used in the reference situation [6].

Consideration should also be given to the format of materials, both print and nonprint, in the reference collection. Specifically, will tools only available in microform or electronic format (e.g., online databases, portable databases on CD-ROM and diskette) be acceptable? Which types of tools will be considered for purchase in print form? In electronic formats? In which other formats? For ready-reference purposes, will access to databases on bibliographic utilities be considered in lieu of purchase for a particular title?

Online and portable electronic formats—sources of both bibliographic information and factual data—can be considered a part of the reference collection and should be included as a possible format for reference access in the collection policy statement. It could be argued that online and portable electronic sources form a separate reference service; however, they are considered here as additional formats for some of the most heavily used reference tools: indexes, abstracts, and drug/chemical sources.

Full-text online searching of a number of journals provides another approach to answering reference queries. Both BRS and DIALOG offer a number of full-text journals and newsletters online, and BRS's Comprehensive Core Medical Library provides the full text to seventeen major medical textbooks and more than seventy-four journals. The AIDS KnowledgeBase, a continuously updated textbook from San Francisco General Hospital, is available for full-text searching both online and on CD-ROM as Compact-Library:AIDS. These provide just two technological advances that are having an impact on reference service and the reference collection development policy. The advent of videodisc storage and retrieval will also change the nature of tools selected for a reference collection; however, as yet, it has not become a familiar format in health sciences libraries' reference collections [7]. Having a well-defined written reference collection development policy will make it easier to fit these new tools and other sources into a collection.

Another area to consider is duplication of materials. Some tools, such as heavily used textbooks, should be considered for both the circulating and reference collections. Also, duplicate copies of heavily used reference books, e.g., medical dictionaries or the *Physicians' Desk Reference (PDR)*, may be needed at the reference desk and in the reference office, in addition to the reference collection. The need for multiple formats in bibliographic tools also needs to be considered.

In the example of a reference collection policy outline [8-11] shown in Table 1-1, consideration of formats and multiple copies are listed separately for illustrative purposes. Alternately, they could be incorporated into section V under each specific category.

Table 1-1. Outline for a Reference Collection Policy

I. Introduction
    A. History of the policy
        1. Date of the original formulation
        2. Authority establishing the policy
    B. Present revision of the policy with the date of approval

II. Objectives of the reference collection
    A. Purpose of the collection
    B. Clientele served

III. Scope of the reference collection related to:
    A. User information needs
    B. Subject coverage in relation to the overall collection policy of the library
    C. Depth of collection of materials by subject
    D. Subjects outside the scope of the collection

IV. Physical size of the collection

V. Categories of reference materials
    A. Information on persons, organizations, or institutions
        1. Directories of persons—biographical directories
        2. Directories of organizations
        3. Telephone directories
    B. Factual data
        1. Dictionaries
            a. General English-language
            b. Subject
            c. Foreign-language/polyglot
        2. Encyclopedias
        3. Handbooks
        4. Drug/chemical sources
        5. Statistical sources
        6. Legislation, regulations
            a. Federal
            b. State
            c. Local
        7. Catalogs
            a. Educational institutions
            b. Commercial products, including laboratory equipment and supplies

Table 1-1 (cont.)

    8. Manuals and guides
      a. Writing and style manuals
      b. Online search manuals
    9. Indexes, abstracts, and bibliographies
    10. Lists of meetings

  C. Union lists and catalogs
    1. Book catalogs
    2. Serial sources
      a. Union lists
      b. Abbreviations lists, lists of journals indexed or abstracted
        (included by indexing and abstracting services)
    3. Audiovisual software sources
      a. Catalogs from producers
      b. Union lists
    4. Translation sources
  D. Textbooks and histories
  E. Ephemeral and pamphlet materials

VI. Format
  A. Print
  B. Nonprint
    1. Microcomputer software
    2. CD-ROMs, diskettes
    3. Microforms
    4. Online databases

VII. Multiple copies
  A. Serials, e.g., *Index Medicus*
    1. Determination of need
    2. Locations: reference, reference office, journal stacks, etc.
  B. Books, e.g., medical dictionary, *PDR*
    1. Determination of need
    2. Locations: reference stacks, reference desk, reference office,
      reading room(s), etc.
  C. Online search tools
    1. Determination of need
    2. Locations: reference office, terminal/PC location(s), reference
      desk, etc.

Writing the reference collection policy should not be considered an academic exercise. It is a concrete means by which a collection can be measured and developed. It can also be used to orient and train new librarians and Reference staff about the collection and the types of materials needed to serve the library's clientele. The outline in Table 1-1 provides a framework for developing a policy [12] (*see also* Appendix 1). However, a policy, like a collection, must be reviewed regularly to determine if it fulfills the goals of maintaining a vital reference collection. The policy should be considered a creative tool.

Along with the collection development policy for reference, there should be a sensible weeding and retention policy. Many reference tools come out in new editions at regular intervals—annually or biennially, for example. It would be impossible to maintain a usable reference collection if all these editions were kept in the reference collection. Unlike weeding for the general collection, in which materials are discarded or offered on exchange to other libraries, a reference weeding policy has the option of retiring earlier editions of reference tools to the general circulating collection. Of course, duplicate copies could be withdrawn; two copies of the 1991 *American Hospital Association Guide to the Health Care Field* in the circulating collection would not be sensible when there are two copies of the current edition in the reference collection. In this example, one copy is sufficient for comparative or historical purposes.

In some instances, however, it is useful to keep more than one edition of a tool in the reference collection. For example, when the latest edition of a reference book drops a section and the only source of the information is the earlier edition of the book, it is advisable to keep both editions on reference.

A reference collection weeding policy could be outlined as shown in Table 1-2.

Although a separate outline for a weeding policy is presented here, retention information could be easily incorporated into a reference collection policy for each category of reference tool. See Appendix 1 for an example of a combined selection-retention policy statement.

In practice, most libraries rely on the serial nature of many reference tools to keep the collection current and "weeded," withdrawing an earlier edition or sending it to the general collection when a new edition appears. In fact, they have a continuous weeding process. However, there are many reference materials that are not necessarily updated on a regular basis to trigger the weeding process. To maintain a current relevant collection, it is advisable to have an annual or biennial review of the reference collection, following the guidelines in the reference collection policy. Other factors that prompt weeding include space limitations, material in disrepair, and subjects no longer useful for reference purposes. Adalian and Rockman recom-

Table 1-2. Outline for a Reference Weeding Policy

I. Introduction
  A. History of the policy
    1. Date of original formulation
    2. Authority establishing the policy
  B. Present revision of the policy with the date of approval

II. Purpose of the policy

III. Retention policy
  (To be coordinated with the overall collection development policy for areas in which exhaustive collections or archival material would always be kept.)
  A. Only the latest edition is kept in library on reference (primary materials that supersede themselves)
    1. Online manuals
    2. Holdings lists of individual libraries
    3. Pamphlets
    4. Catalogs (college, audiovisual producers, equipment, etc.)
  B. Latest edition kept on reference, earlier editions in circulating collection

    1. Any category A materials (above) found to be unique and worth retaining in the collection for historical or research purposes
    2. Dictionaries
    3. Directories
    4. Handbooks
    5. Drug sources
    6. Textbooks
    7. Encyclopedias
    8. Writing and style manuals
    9. Book catalogs
  C. Earlier editions kept on reference as usefulness to reference and available space permit
    1. Any category B materials (above) containing unique information found useful to reference
    2. Indexing and abstracting services
    3. Bibliographies
    4. Statistical sources
    5. Union lists and serials sources
    6. Translation sources
    7. Lists of meetings

mend a title-by-title review of reference materials and identify nine objectives for such a review.

1. To serve as an inventory of the reference collection, identifying missing titles and volumes.
2. To serve as a means of purging the reference collection of seldom-used or obsolete books, which would be transferred to either a storage facility or the circulating collection, or eliminated from the library entirely.
3. To monitor standing orders which require claim action by the serials department.
4. To determine the appropriateness of all standing orders to see if only the latest edition or all volumes of a continuation should be kept in the reference department.
5. To ascertain whether a standing order should be placed for a serial title that was held in the collection but for which no standing order existed.
6. To determine if a later edition of a title not published on a regular basis is needed in the reference collection.
7. To identify gaps in the reference collection.
8. To identify and order a current title comparable in subject to an earlier title of which no updated edition is available.
9. To serve as a continuing education vehicle for the reference librarians, by which they could become better acquainted with the strengths and weaknesses of the collection, and therefore more proficient in selecting titles for, and retrieving information from it [13].

Access to the tools in the reference collection is generally through the public catalog. Online public access catalogs (OPACs) provide copy location information for those libraries that have automated their holdings records and provide a means of identifying those materials in the reference collection. For libraries still using a card catalog, a stamped note or plastic overlay on the card will indicate that an item is in the reference collection, or add "also in reference" on the catalog card for items that are in the general collection and duplicated in reference. Larger libraries may have a separate reference catalog or reference shelflist for access to the reference collection alone. However, in libraries where the reference collection is small, items in the general collection may be used more frequently than in large libraries to answer clients' questions; in this case, access to all items, including reference materials, through a single public catalog would be preferable.

Organization of the Reference Collection

How should the reference collection be organized? There are varying schools of thought on this subject. A reference collection consists of both monographic and serial publications. The monographic collection will probably be classified by means of the National Library of Medicine's (NLM) classification system or some other method. The serial collection may or may not be classified; many libraries prefer to arrange their serials alphabetically. Some additional questions may arise concerning serials in the reference collection: Are reference serials to be classified or arranged alphabetically? Which items are considered serials in reference—just the indexes and abstracts, or all serial publications?

If an entirely classified arrangement is chosen, the collection is usually shelved by classified (subject) arrangement, regardless of the type or format of the material. An exception is often made for indexes and abstracts, which are arranged on index tables for ease of use. The NLM classification scheme allows for format division within subject categories. For example, directories are indicated by "22":

W 22	general medical
WU 22	dental
WX 22	hospital

and dictionaries by "13":

W 13	general medical
WM 13	psychiatry
WY 13	nursing

thus affording a degree of form arrangement within a broader subject arrangement.

A modification of the classified arrangement can also be used, in which the monographic collection is classified and arranged by call number but the serial publications are arranged alphabetically and not classified. These are primarily indexes and abstracts, but can also include other serial publications (e.g., *World Meetings, Unlisted Drugs, Vital and Health Statistics*) usually found in a reference collection. In practice, some libraries classify reference serials, others leave them alphabetically arranged, and others group them chronologically, as is frequently done with the medical indexes, *Index Medicus*, and its predecessors. One real problem with the alphabetically arranged serials collection arises when the title of a work changes, separating consecutive volumes of the work.

The monographic reference collection, while classified, may not always be arranged strictly by call number. Some reference departments prefer an arrangement by form categories [14-15] (*see* Reference Categories list below) in which all dictionaries, directories, handbooks, and so on are shelved together. These categories are not arranged just by form, however.

Some provide subject groupings, such as "drug lists," which include handbooks, dictionaries, manuals, etc., on the subject. Other libraries have a combination of a classified arrangement with a form arrangement for heavily used items such as dictionaries, directories, textbooks, and college catalogs. When such arrangements are used, proper labeling of the public catalog or holdings statements in an online catalog and of the reference collection is essential to guide the user to the location of the material in the reference area. Pizer and Walker caution that "such a reorganization of the collection, however, required additional...files to indicate shelf position and that makes the user dependent upon library staff to point out locations" [16].

Reference Categories

1. Dictionaries (medical and other subjects; English and foreign; also includes nomenclature, terminology, and quotation lists)
2. Manuals and guides (style manuals, writing guides, programmed textbooks on medical terminology, legal and ethical manuals)
3. Almanacs and statistical compilations (includes all reference material on statistics)
4. Subject handbooks (data books such as *Handbook of Chemistry and Physics, Biology Data Handbook, Handbook of Clinical Laboratory Data*)
5. Drug lists (all reference materials on drugs, including manuals, dictionaries, and handbooks)
6. Biographical directories (includes all reference materials listing people)
7. Directories (includes listings of institutions, organizations, scholarships, educational programs, agencies)
8. Geographical atlases (includes geographical materials such as *Webster's Atlas and Zip Code Directory, Hotel and Motel Red Book*)
9. Encyclopedias and encyclopedic works (such as *Encyclopedia Britannica, Handbook of Experimental Pharmacology, Practice of Medicine*)
10. Library information (includes directories, handbooks, and manuals in the field of library science)
11. Bibliographies and histories (includes selected bibliographies in the health sciences, histories of medicine, and nonprint media)
12. Serial information (includes union catalogs, abbreviations lists, directories of periodicals such as *Ulrich's International Periodicals Directory*)
13. Book catalogs (includes listings of books such as *Books in Print, National Library of Medicine Current Catalog, Cumulative Book Index*)
14. Lists of meetings and translations (such as *Technical Translations Index, World Meetings: United States and Canada, Annual International Congress Calendar*)

Whatever arrangement is chosen, consideration must be made for ease of use by the library user as well as the reference librarian. Jeuell, in presenting an arrangement by categories, argues that arrangement by form increases the retrievability of information from the collection, because clients frequently want a *type* of information (e.g., biographical) but may not know the subject area in which to look. A classified arrangement would require looking for biographies in several subject areas. She concludes

> Form arrangement results in efficient use of the monographic collection by making it more retrievable, in terms of the patron's information needs, than a straight call number arrangement. Arrangement by form takes into account that some vital information might be missing from a reference question, and that many patrons use a monographic reference collection by browsing through a group of similar books such as biographical directories, rather than looking for a subject or for a specific title in the card catalog [17].

On the other hand, arrangement by form can lead to arbitrary placement of books in a category. Some items are neither strictly handbooks, statistical sources, nor directories. In which category should they be placed? How efficiently is the patron then served? Subject arrangement (classified) does scatter similar forms of publications; however, it increases "browsabililty" within a field of interest—ophthalmology, hospitals, nursing, etc.

Of course there are times when form arrangement would have its advantages and times when subject arrangement would be more advantageous. The arrangement chosen will depend on how the reference staff uses the collection and how it perceives the majority of clients use the collection—by form or by subject.

Recent discussion over the medical libraries discussion list, MEDLIB-L, on the Internet revealed that this is an issue still being debated among health sciences librarians. The experience at McMaster University Health Sciences Library provides a lesson for any library contemplating a change.

> Some years ago, our small-to-medium Reference Collection was arranged so as to group all the dictionaries together, all the encyclopedias, all the handbooks, all the style manuals, on the theory that it would be easier for the patrons to find the item they wanted if all they could remember was that it was a dictionary...or whatever...It did not work very well in our quite small collection, and I fear that it would be much worse in a larger collection. You could no longer rely on your years of experience in locating material by subject throughout the NLM classification because the order in which books were found on the shelf had been totally altered. A

new classification had to be learned; it was devised to be simple, but it was new, and didn't seem to be as "natural" either to users or staff as had been hoped it would be....We had a re-arranged shelf list, and a key to show us if we knew the call number where to find it on the re-arranged shelves, but it took longer because there were two look-ups rather than one!

The patrons didn't seem to reap great benefit from the rearrangement, either...some intuited quite easily where to locate what they wanted, but others were simply not on that wave length at all! The catalogue was of no use to them because the translation tool was at the Reference Desk, intended mainly for staff use, since it was assumed that the patrons would find the new shelf arrangement easy-to-use....

We went back to shelving according to the NLM classification about five years ago simply because our effort to make using the Reference Collection simpler didn't work....We went back to NLM shelving in the Reference Collection for the sake of consistency and because it actually promoted the likelihood that patrons would find what they wanted in Reference. They were more familiar with it than our new scheme! [18]

The physical arrangement of the collection will also depend to a great extent on the space available. Whether the "ideal" arrangement is considered to be by form categories, classified, or a combination of classified and alphabetic, the actual arrangement may be determined by where the collection can be housed. There may not be enough room for all the indexes and abstracts to fit on index tables. Which ones should be arranged on the tables? In what order? Obviously, *Index Medicus* should be there, but volumes for how many years should be kept at this access point?

Should the monographic reference collection and other reference serials be near the reference desk? If not, should the collection be split to provide quick access to the most frequently used tools? Or should the collection have duplicate copies of heavily used items, one set for the reference stacks and one for the reference desk or "Ready Reference"? Is there space available at the desk? Will space constraints determine the use of form arrangement versus classified subject arrangement?

If space is at a premium, should microform (film or fiche) be considered as the primary format for some tools? If so, which ones? *Chemical Abstracts*? Telephone books? Medical school and college catalogs? How are these to be arranged in relation to the other tools in the collection? Is there space for microform readers in the reference area? How many are needed?

With more and more reference tools becoming available in electronic format, the place for this format must also be considered. Will the reference area have one microcomputer and CD-ROM player for any and all electronic reference tools in the collection, both bibliographic and non-bibliographic? Or will there be a work station for each reference tool available in this format? Will bibliographic or nonbibliographic CD-ROMs be on a network? If so, how many stations will be provided? Will remote, dial-up access be available? If yes, how many ports will be available for remote access? How will the reference area be arranged for both client and staff use of these tools? What will their proximity be to the reference desk and print reference collection?

These are just a few of the questions that must be considered in deciding how to arrange a reference collection. There is no perfect answer—each library has a collection unique in size and content, based on the use and reference demands of its clientele. How the collection is arranged should be determined by these use and reference patterns, to maximize efficient use of the collection within the space constraints of the building. Easy, logical access to the collection by the clients and staff should be the goal for a collection's organization and physical arrangement.

SELECTION OF MATERIALS

Maintaining the collection is an ongoing process. Current addresses, telephone numbers, statistical data, etc., are often the information sought from a reference tool. To provide such information, it is important to have the latest available edition of a tool in the collection. There are several ways to keep current. These include (1) publishers' announcements; (2) acquisitions lists of other health sciences libraries; and (3) online cataloging files. Based on the author's recent survey, health sciences librarians from both academic and hospital libraries rely most heavily on publishers' announcements for identifying new editions of reference books. However, many libraries rely on approval plans for receipt of new editions and identification of potential new titles for Reference. Having a book in hand to evaluate before purchase is highly valued. The survey also indicated that the Brandon/Hill lists, vendors, or publishers, newsletters, and the American College of Physicians' *Library for Internists* are also used for selection of reference materials.

Acquisitions lists from other libraries were mentioned as being helpful. As Eakin points out, these are useful because "sources of information about less common reference tools may be obscure or may more easily be missed. Another exception may be in areas of special interest, and it may be worthwhile to check the acquisitions list of a particular library for a single subject..." [19].

While not limited to reviewing reference books, health sciences journals provide regular book review sections, e.g., *Annals of Internal Medicine's* "The

Literature of Note" and *JAMA*'s "Books, Journals, Software." These journals and others are available in full text online through such services as BRS' Comprehensive Core Medical Library (CCML), MEDTEXT, and Health Periodicals Database where the book reviews are searchable [20].

Many reference books are serials that appear in new editions annually. Academic libraries, more than hospital libraries, rely on standing orders with publishers or vendors for these titles, thus being assured of timely receipt of new editions or volumes. However, the convenience of approval plans and standing orders does not preclude the librarian's responsibility for final selection decisions. "Human involvement in collection decision making is essential for developing user-responsive collections" [21].

When new reference tools are selected, the guidelines from the reference collection policy should be followed. Is the tool going to provide new information? Does it duplicate information available in other tools? If so, is the information in a more easily retrievable format, making this new tool a desirable acquisition? Often this information is not discernible from a publisher's announcement. If the reference tool is not available through the approval plan, it may be advisable to wait until a review is published in a library journal such as the *Bulletin of the Medical Library Association* or *Medical Reference Services Quarterly*. These two sources were most frequently cited in the survey as having helpful reviews for selecting reference materials. Other sources for reviews of new tools are the various regional medical library newsletters. These are aimed at hospital and small academic libraries and can provide guides for such collections.

Using the cataloging databases as aids in selection can also be helpful. Both the National Library of Medicine's CATLINE (CATalog onLINE) file and the Online Computer Library Center (OCLC) database can be used in ascertaining the latest edition of a particular work. CATLINE is particularly useful in identifying new material in a subject field, while SERLINE (SERials onLINE) can provide similar information for periodicals. In practice, CATLINE is an underutilized source for identifying relevant reference tools, with only a few of the surveyed libraries indicating that they are using CATLINE for this purpose. However, a number of libraries indicated the usefulness of the National Library of Medicine's *Current Catalog Proof Sheets (CCPS)*, distributed by the Medical Library Association. Unfortunately, NLM is discontinuing its Reference Notes in CATLINE because of low use by libraries, and the Medical Library Association will cease distribution of the NLM *Current Catalog Proof Sheets* in 1993. However, the NLM Locator, that library's catalog via the Internet, should readily provide access to this information for many libraries.

Selection of materials for the reference collection is generally a team effort. While in smaller libraries the library director is responsible for selection, all staff who use the collection are encouraged to identify titles and make recommendations. In larger libraries, public services staff members are all expected to contribute suggestions or make recommendations, with the ultimate decisions left to the library director or the head of public services or the head of collections/acquisitions or a combination of all the above. In some larger libraries, one of the Reference librarians is responsible for identifying appropriate materials for the Reference collection and then soliciting comments from fellow librarians.

When it comes to selection of electronic reference sources, the decisions are generally made by a broader group, including the library director, the head of systems, the head of audiovisuals, and the head of public services/reference. In larger institutions and when the health sciences library has close ties to the general campus, such decisions are made by campus-wide committees. This is especially true for databases mounted locally on minicomputers or on shared local area network (LAN) facilities.

Criteria for Evaluating New Material

Once identified, these tools need to be measured against the existing collections in accordance with the reference collection development policy. Criteria for evaluating new materials include [22-23]:

1. Significance and usefulness of the title.
2. Authority and reputation of the author, publisher or database producer.
3. Age and currency of the work and its contents.
4. Favorable reviews in the professional literature.
5. Inclusion of the title in reference guides.
6. Difficulty level of the contents.
7. Language of the publication.
8. Price of the publication or database in relation to
   a. availability of the information contained,
   b. quality and physical production of the title, and
   c. length of use.
9. Anticipated frequency of use (judge in relation to cost, available format[s], and space).
10. Appropriate format (print vs microform vs electronic).

The above criteria are also useful for maintaining and weeding the existing collection. Materials in some areas are particularly difficult to keep current. Directories of specialized societies are often published once, then abandoned or published sporadically. Statistical sources can also be a problem. A study may be done once, then never updated. Keeping an eye out for a useful new reference tool is aided by having a good working knowledge of the Reference collection and the policy guidelines. When looking at specific reference tools, librarians use a combination of measures for evaluation, with a definite focus on their usefulness for the audience who will use these tools. The ideal combination of criteria includes authority of the material in scope and subject coverage which presents the information in an easy-to-read format. Because budgets are frequently limited, librarians aim to select materials that are most appropriate to *their* particular library's collection and clientele. They look for new tools that will fill gaps in their collection. Other evaluative criteria used for selecting reference materials include good indexes, uniqueness of presentation, clear tables and illustrations, logical organization, and clarity of presentation.

Criteria for selecting electronic reference sources require the same scope and subject coverage considerations used for print sources. Additional factors to consider include search features offered, single vendor for consistent format when offering multiple databases, and price. Tenopir outlines evaluation criteria for both online sources and CD-ROMs.

For online sources consider

1. Connecting to the system.
2. Search language.
3. Effectiveness of search program.
4. Contents quality.
5. Search aids.

For CD-ROMs consider

1. Scope
2. Content
3. Quality
4. Accessibility [24].

Library Journal's survey of public, academic, and special libraries use of CD-ROMs noted that "the most important criterion in the selection of a CD-ROM database was...accuracy/authority. Ease of use and value for cost came in second and third, and most of the libraries felt that 'depth and breadth' of the product (scope or years and titles covered) were important" [25].

Because most of the electronic reference sources also have print counterparts, a decision must be made as to whether to duplicate formats. Often electronic formats are only available for lease; consequently, libraries are reluctant to give up print versions when their collections serve an archival role. Often producers and vendors will give a "discount" price for the electronic format when a library also has a subscription to the print version, providing additional incentive to duplicate formats. In addition, the electronic formats are not, as yet, considered archival by library archivists.

Electronic versions of bibliographic sources have been widely accepted by health sciences libraries, with print versions also maintained for the most heavily used indexing and abstracting services. However, the lesser-used sources for a particular library are increasingly being made available in electronic format only and often for the first time in health sciences libraries, e.g., Wilson indexes and ERIC. Academic libraries frequently have LAN and locally mounted networks of databases that provide campuswide access to a number of sources not available in the health sciences library, while hospital libraries are forming consortia or affiliating with academic libraries to make such sources available to their clientele.

The nonbibliographic electronic sources, such as Micromedex CCIS, CompactLibrary:AIDS, and AMA-FRIEDA, have been well received by reference librarians. However, most other nonbibliographic electronic reference sources have not been well received, based on comments made in the author's survey. Print versions are considered more useful for quick look-up, and ready reference requires this accessibility. When electronic formats are provided, the print version is also maintained in the collection. The cost of maintaining duplicate versions of these materials, coupled with the cost of providing and maintaining an adequate range of equipment on which to mount the electronic versions, appears to be prohibitive for many libraries. In lieu of purchase or lease of electronic reference tools, some libraries are providing direct client access to a number of vendor services, such as NLM's GRATEFUL MED, BRS Colleague, PaperChase, and DIALOG Medical Connection. Smaller libraries are providing online ready reference from nonbibliographic reference sources, e.g., *Encyclopedia of Associations*, that they do not have in print [26]. With the growing use of Internet connections to both commercial vendors and alternative sources such as bulletin boards, discussion lists, and specialized databases, libraries are extending their reference services even further. Tenopir sums it up best in a recent *Library Journal* article: "Commercial online, alternative online, Internet, CD-ROM, or locally loaded databases—which are most important? ALL are important...since each has its own unique advantages, all libraries should be offering some combination of services...some combination is possible and necessary for every library" [27].

Regardless of library size, about 5%-8% of the budget is spent on reference materials [28]. Few libraries maintain a separate budget for reference materials, with the serial publications for reference funded most often through the library's serials budget. Many libraries also fund electronic reference tools through the serials budget as well. Sources other than the regular acquisitions budget (grants, gifts, and endowments) are frequently used to fund expensive electronic reference tools.

Additional funding outside the acquisitions budget must be sought to purchase and maintain the equipment needed to use electronic sources. Funding sources vary among libraries. Some are able to fund such purchases from regular equipment budgets, while other libraries must seek alternative funding, such as capital requests, grants, and gifts and endowments. Many libraries use a combination of funding sources.

The purpose of this chapter has not been to provide answers. It is intended to present the issues relating to the way a reference collection is developed, organized, and maintained. There are many factors to consider. The questions raised here are meant to lead to thoughtful consideration of how best to organize a new collection or an existing one, or to assess how an existing collection came to be the way it is. The important question is, How can the collection best serve the user?

REFERENCES

1. Reference collection development: a bibliography. Neeley J, ed. Chicago: Reference and Adult Service Division, American Library Association, 1991.

2. Beatty WK. Technical processes: Part 1. Selection, acquisition, and weeding. In: Annan GL and Felter JW, eds. Handbook of medical library practice. 3d. ed. Chicago: Medical Library Association, 1970:71-92.

3. National Library of Medicine, Technical Services Division. Collection Development Manual of the National Library of Medicine. Bethesda, MD: National Library of Medicine, 1985.

4. Eakin D. Health science library materials: collection development. In: Darling L, ed. Handbook of medical library practice, 4th ed. Chicago: Medical Library Association, 1983:36-8.

5. Beatty, Technical Processes:73.

6. See: England JW. Library Collection development policy. Philadelphia, Pennsylvania. In: Collection development policies for college libraries. Chicago: American Library Association, 1989:68-83. (Clip Note No. 11)

7. Based on responses to the author's survey on reference collection development practices in academic health sciences libraries and hospital libraries, Fall 1991. (unpublished)

8. Ibid.:73-4.

9. Houston Academy of Medicine, Texas Medical Center Library Collection development policy. 1978 Apr (Unpublished manuscript).

10. Kwan JK. Reverence collection policy, Los Angeles: UCLA Biomedical Library, 1983 Aug (Unpublished manuscript).

11. Lehocky B. Academic reference collection development policy statement. Arlington, VA: ERIC Document Reproduction Service, 1979. ERIC document ED 190160.

12. See: Other criteria: Thomas Jefferson Univ; Johns Hopkins Univ. In: Collection Development Policies for Health Sciences Libraries, Morse DH and Richards DT compilers. Chicago: Medical Library Association, 1992:128-37. (MLA DocKit #3)

13. Adalian PT, Jr., Rockman IF. Title-by-title review in reference collection development. Ref Serv Rev 1984 Winter; 12:86.

14. Jeuell CA. The reorganization of a monographic reference collection. Bull Med Lib Assoc, 1976 July;64:293-8.

15. Truelson SD, Jr. The totally organized reference collection. Bull Med Lib Assoc 1976 July;50:184-7.

16. Pizer IR, Walker WD. Physical access to resources: The reference collection. In: Darling L, ed. Handbook of medical library practice, 4th ed. V. 1. Chicago: Medical Library Association, 1982:25.

17. Jeuell. Reorganization of reference collection:298.

18. Flemming T. Arrangement of reference collection. Message to: Multiple recipients of list MEDLIB-L. In: MEDLIB-L@uvbm.cc.buffalo.edu [discussion list]. Start N, list owner. [Buffalo]: [State University of New York at Buffalo]. 1992 June 18. [62 lines]

19. Eakin. Health sciences library materials:46-7.

20. See: Van Camp AJ. Finding health sciences books and book reviews online. Online 1993 May;17:120-123.

21. Hattendorf LC. The art of reference collection development. RQ 1989;29(2):220.

22. Kwan, Reference collection policy:23-4.

23. Lehocky, Academic reference collection development policy:61.

24. Tenopir C. Evaluation criteria for online, CD-ROM. Lib J 1992 1 March;117:68.

25. Berry J. CD-ROM: the medium of the moment. Libr J 1992 1 Feb; 117:46.

26. Author's survey, Fall 1991. (unpublished)

27. Tenopir C. Online Databases: choices for electronic reference. Lib J 1993 1 July; 118:53.

28. Author's survey, Fall 1991. (unpublished)

READINGS

Bryant B, ed., Guide for written collection policy statements. Chicago: American Library Association, 1989. (Collection Management and Development Guides, No. 3)

Coleman K, Dickinson P. Drafting a reference collection policy. Coll Res Libr 1977 May;38:227-33.

Desmarias N, ed. CD-ROM local area networks: a users guide. Westport, CT: Meckler Publishing, 1991.

Jasco P. CD-ROM software, dataware, and hardware: evaluation, selection, and installation. Englewood, CO: Libraries Unlimited, 1992.

Kroll R. The place of reference collection development in the organizational structure of the library. RQ 1985;25(1):96-100.

La Guardia C. Electronic databases: will old collection development policies still work? Online 1992 July;16:60-63.

Management of CD-ROM datbases in ARL libraries. Washington, DC: Association of Research Libraries, 1990. (OMS SpecKit no. 169)

Pfaffenberger B. Democratizing information: online databases and the rise of end-user searching. Boston: G.K. Hall, 1990.

Pierce SJ, ed. Weeding and maintenance of reference collections. New York: Haworth Press, 1990.

Reference collection development: a bibliography: a project of the Reference Collection Development and Evaluation Section, Reference and Adult Services. Chicago: Reference and Adult Services Division, American Library Association, 1991.

Teich S, Righetti MA, eds. Collection development in the health sciences: building a basic reference collection. 2d ed. Portland: Oregon Health Sciences Libraries Association, 1987.

Loren D. Carlson Health Sciences Library Reference Collection Policy

August 1992

INTRODUCTION

The reference collection is a primary resource within the library for identifying sources of information as well as answering factual and bibliographic questions. The reference collection differs from the circulating collection; materials in the reference collection are consulted for specific information rather than read from beginning to end. To assure that these materials are available for immediate use, the reference collection is separated from the circulating collection, housed in an easily accessible area, and made non-circulating.

LIBRARY CLIENTELE

Primary library clientele include faculty, research staff, and graduate students in the School of Medicine and the School of Veterinary Medicine. The library also serves faculty, research staff, graduate students, and undergraduates in fields related to human medicine, veterinary medicine, and the health and life sciences.

SCOPE OF THE COLLECTION

The scope of the collection encompasses human medicine, veterinary medicine, and the health and life sciences. Subject coverage of the reference collection primarily reflects the research and educational goals of the UCD School of Medicine and the School of Veterinary Medicine. However, reference materials in a number of secondary areas are included in the collection due to the interdisciplinary nature of these fields.

Materials within the field of veterinary medicine are collected at the comprehensive level; within the field of human medicine at the research level; and within secondary areas at the instructional support level.

SELECTION METHODS

Reference librarians use a variety of tools in selecting materials for the reference collection, including the MELVYL online catalog, OCLC, faculty recommendations, book reviews, library newsletters, and publishers' announcements. Since our subscription to the *National Library of Medicine Current Catalog Proof Sheets* was cancelled in 1992, implementation of a CATLINE SDI is being considered as an aid in the selection of reference materials.

SELECTION CRITERIA

Major criteria for evaluating new materials include the significance and usefulness of the title; authority and reputation of the author(s), editor(s), and contributors; reputation of the publisher or database producer; favorable reviews in professional literature; format; and price of the publication or database. With the exception of foreign-language dictionaries, foreign-language materials are not selected for the reference collection.

RETENTION POLICY

The retention policy includes the following five categories for weeding reference materials:

Category A: The latest edition is retained on reference; earlier editions are discarded
Category B: The latest edition is retained on reference; earlier editions are retired to the circulating collection
Category C: The latest as well as earlier editions are retained on reference
Category D: The next-to-the-latest edition is retained on reference (the latest edition is held at another UCD library); earlier editions are discarded
Category E: The next-to-the-latest edition is retained on reference (the latest edition is held at another UCD library); earlier editions are retired to the circulating collection

FORMAT

Reference materials will generally be purchased in print format. Non-print formats may be selected for certain categories of materials, including indexes, abstracts, drug/chemical sources, and serial sources.

Indexes and abstracts are often more convenient to use in online or CD-ROM format. Heavily used indexes and abstracts may be leased in online or CD-ROM format as well as purchased in print format. Less heavily used products may be leased in online or CD-ROM format or purchased in print format. And finally, databases may be leased for use on the UC Davis CD-ROM network when the subject content is appropriate for multiple library locations.

Updates of drug/chemical sources may be issued in microfiche format by the publisher. Microfiche format may also be used for serial sources, such as union lists, as an economic and space-saving measure. However, print format is generally preferred to microfiche format due to the inconvenient and difficult nature of microfiche products.

MULTIPLE COPIES

Multiple copies of certain heavily used reference materials may be purchased for the circulating collection, reserves collection, reference desk, or online room, as well as the reference collection. However, unless otherwise specified, one copy of each item within the following categories will be kept in the reference collection.

CATEGORIES OF REFERENCE MATERIALS

A. Information on persons, organizations, or institutions
  1. Directories of education
     Scope: Educational directories of professional schools within the scope of the collection; general undergraduate educational directories
     Retention: Category A or B; earlier editions are generally discarded; earlier editions within the scope of the collection containing detailed information on programs or representing a substantial body of work from a major association are retired to the circulating collection
     Format: Print
  2. Directories of funding sources
     Scope: Current materials on funding sources and research within the scope of the collection
     Retention: Category A or B; earlier editions are generally discarded; earlier editions containing detailed award information are retired to the circulating collection
     Format: Print

3. Directories of libraries
   Scope: Directories of libraries, librarians, and library associations
   Retention: Category A or B; earlier editions of directories of libraries and librarians are generally discarded; directories of health sciences libraries are retired to the circulating collection
   Format: Print
4. Directories of organizations and institutions
   Scope: Directories of organizations and institutions within the scope of the collection; major interdisciplinary directories
   Retention: Category A, B or D; the latest editions of directories within the scope of the collection are retained on reference; earlier editions containing information in core fields for this library are retired to the circulating collection (e.g., *AVMA Directory*); only the next to the latest editions of certain interdisciplinary directories are retained on reference (e.g., *Thomas Register*)
   Format: Print
5. Directories of persons/biographical directories
   Scope: Directories of persons/biographical directories within the scope of the collection; major interdisciplinary directories
   Retention: Category A or B; earlier editions are generally discarded; earlier editions containing detailed biographical information are retired to the circulating collection
   Format: Print
6. Directories of services
   Scope: Directories of medical or veterinary services; patient referral sources
   Retention: Category A or B; earlier editions are selectively retired to the circulating collection
   Format: Print
7. Telephone directories
   Scope: Current telephone directories for selected northern California communities
   Retention: Category A
   Format: Print
B. Factual data
   1. Authority lists
      Scope: National Library of Medicine and Library of Congress subject headings
      Retention: Category A
      Format: Print
      Multiple Copies: Reference Desk, Reference Collection, Online Room
   2. Bibliographies
      Scope: National Library of Medicine subject bibliographies; other

selected bibliographies on topics within the scope of the collection
Retention: Category C
Format: Print
3. Dictionaries
   (a) English-language dictionaries
   Scope: Small collection of authoritative general dictionaries; extensive collection of authoritative specialized dictionaries in subject areas within the scope of the collection
   Retention: Category B
   Format: Print
   Multiple Copies: Reference Desk, Reference Collection, Online Room (specialized dictionaries)
   (b) Foreign-language dictionaries
   Scope: Small collection of foreign-language general dictionaries; small collection of specialized dictionaries in subject areas within the scope of the collection; European languages, Russian, Chinese, and Japanese; foreign/English or English/foreign format
   Retention: Category B
   Format: Print
4. Drug/chemical sources
   Scope: Current national and international human and veterinary drug information sources
   Retention: Category B
   Format: Print, Microfiche
5. Encyclopedias
   Scope: One authoritative general encyclopedia; specialized encyclopedias in subject areas within the scope of the collection
   Retention: Category B
   Format: Print
6. General reference sources
   Scope: General reference sources, such as almanacs, books of quotations, and fact books
   Retention: Category A or B; earlier editions are selectively retired to the circulating collection
   Format: Print
7. Geographic sources
   Scope: Small collection of U.S. and world atlases; current maps of the local area; campus maps
   Retention: Category A or B; superceded atlases are retired to the circulating collection; earlier editions of local area and campus maps are discarded
   Format: Print

8. Government documents and technical reports sources
Scope: Sources for identifying government documents and technical reports
Retention: Category C
Format: Print

9. Guides to the literature
Scope: Authoritative guides to literature within the scope of the collection
Retention: Category B
Format: Print

10. Handbooks
Scope: Current authoritative handbooks on topics within the scope of the collection
Retention: Category B
Format: Print

11. Indexes and abstracts
Scope: Major indexes and abstracts within the scope of the collection
Retention: Category C
Format: Print, CD-ROM, Online Databases

12. Legislation and regulations
Scope: Basic sources on federal, state, and local government organizations; detailed information on health-related governmental agencies; laws relating to the practice of health professionals
Retention: Category B
Format: Print

13. Licensure and certification
Scope: Current materials on the licensure and certification of health professionals
Retention: Category B
Format: Print

14. Meetings
Scope: Sources for identifying scientific and medical meetings at international, national, and local levels; materials useful for identifying publications resulting from these meetings
Retention: Category C; sources for identifying scientific and medical meetings are retained on reference for five years, earlier editions are discarded
Format: Print

15. Monograph sources
Scope: Sources of information on monographic materials for verification and publication information
Retention: Category A
Format: Print

16. Nomenclature sources
Scope: Authoritative sources on the classification of organisms (biological taxonomy) and disease nomenclature (veterinary and medical nomenclature)
Retention: Category B
Format: Print

17. Popular literature
Scope: Small collection of clearly written, authoritative medical sources written for the general public
Retention: Category B
Format: Print

18. Standards
Scope: Standards relating to the health care and chemical/pharmaceutical industries
Retention: Category B
Format: Print

19. Statistical sources
Scope: Current general statistical sources; specialized statistical sources within the scope of the collection
Retention: Category B
Format: Print

20. Writing and style manuals
Scope: Authoritative writing and style manuals; specialized writing and style manuals in fields relevant to the scope of the collection
Retention: Category B
Format: Print

C. Union lists and catalogs

1. Book catalogs
Scope: Catalogs of libraries having significant subject collections relevant to human medicine, veterinary medicine, and the health and life sciences
Retention: Category A or C; book catalogs are generally retained on reference; earlier editions are discarded only if later editions are cumulative
Format: Print

2. Serial sources

(a) Union lists
Scope: Union lists of titles in major or geographically important libraries or library networks
Retention: Category A or C; earlier editions are generally discarded; in a few cases, earlier editions are retained on reference (e.g., *New Serial Titles*)
Format: Print, Microfiche

(b) Journal abbreviations lists
Scope: Sources providing information on serial titles included in abstracting and indexing services; lists of journal abbreviations
Retention: Category A, B or C; earlier editions of sources providing information on serial titles included in abstracting and indexing services are generally retained
Format: Print
Multiple Copies: Reference Desk, Reference Collection, Online Room

3. Translation sources
Scope: Guides to translations including lists of journals translated from cover-to-cover and guides to translations available through government agencies and other translation sources
Retention: Category C
Format: Print

D. Textbooks
Scope: Small collection of the major medical and veterinary textbooks
Retention: Category B
Format: Print
Multiple Copies: Reference Collection, Reserves Collection, Circulating Collection

E. Ancillary reference materials

1. Annual reports
Scope: Annual reports from organizations and institutions within the scope of the collection
Retention: Category A
Format: Print
Location: Pamphlet File

2. Catalogs
(a) Educational institutions
Scope: Catalogs of American colleges and universities; catalogs of medical and allied health professional schools in the United States and foreign countries; catalogs of veterinary schools in the United States and foreign countries; microfiche copies of medical school catalogs
Retention: Category A
Format: Print, Microfiche
Location: Room 110 (AV Room)

(b) Commercial products
Scope: Catalogs listing equipment and supplies used in medical and veterinary research and patient care
Retention: Category A
Format: Print
Location: Reference Collection, Pamphlet File

3. Online search manuals, etc.
   Scope: Current vendor and database manuals, newsletters, and brochures
   Retention: Category A
   Format: Print
   Location: Room 121 (Online Room)
4. Pamphlets
   Scope: Pamphlets and other ephemeral materials within the scope of the collection such as consumer health information materials
   Retention: Category A
   Format: Print
   Location: Pamphlet File
5. Reference information files
   Scope: Handouts and other materials which facilitate reference service
   Retention: Category A
   Format: Print
   Location: Reference Desk

Prepared by: Judith Welsh, Reference Librarian, Carlson Health Sciences Library, University of California, Davis

PART II

Bibliographic Sources

CHAPTER 2

Bibliographic Sources for Monographs

Fred W. Roper

Although the monograph is no longer the primary means of printed communication in the health sciences, it remains an important component of all library collections, and materials for bibliographic control of monographs are an integral part of any reference collection.

The basic purposes of these materials are verification, location, and selection [1].

Verification is the process by which each item of the needed bibliographic elements, such as author, title, place of publication, and collation, is confirmed. Several sources may have to be consulted to verify various bibliographic elements related to one title. The most useful sources are generally those that are comprehensive in scope.

Location refers to the library or other information agency in which a title may be found or the vendor from which it may be purchased. Online bibliographic databases are the primary sources for identifying holding libraries. Trade bibliographies, which are available in both print and electronic formats, are used to determine availability for purchase. They indicate which titles, regardless of age, are still offered for sale.

Because collection development is such an important part of the information professional's work, the *selection* function presupposes bibliographies that indicate materials available in a given subject area, by a particular author, or in a given format. An evaluation of the worth of an item or an indication of its content in the form of an annotation may be found in some bibliographies.

Bibliographies in the health sciences field may perform more than one of these three functions and are likely to contain entries for more than one type of material: monographs, periodicals, government documents, and so on.

CURRENT SOURCES

Current coverage of medical monographs is primarily carried out by the National Library of Medicine (NLM), using the CATLINE database.

2.1 *CATLINE (CATalog onLINE)*. Bethesda, MD, National Library of Medicine.

2.2 *National Library of Medicine Current Catalog*. Bethesda, MD, National Library of Medicine, 1966-1993. Annual cumulations.

CATLINE offers access to the National Library of Medicine's authoritative bibliographic data for more than 700,000 records. It provides complete cataloging information for all serials and monographs cataloged or recataloged by NLM since 1965, as well as cataloging information supplied by several participating libraries. Virtually all of the cataloged titles in the NLM collection, from the 15th century to the present, are included. CATLINE represents the most up-to-date compilation of cataloging information for health sciences materials, with its weekly updating. About 1,500 new records are added each month. NLM's cataloging records are also available through other databases, such as Online Computer Library Center (OCLC) and Research Libraries Information Network (RLIN).

The *National Library of Medicine Current Catalog* is a byproduct of the CATLINE database. It succeeded earlier NLM catalogs that had been printed as supplements to the Library of Congress (LC) catalogs from 1948 to 1965. Although the *Current Catalog* ceased publication with the 1993 annual cumulation, it continues to be useful for verifying bibliographic citations.

Both monographs and serials are included, with a separate subject and main entry section for each type of material. The full citation is found only under the main entry in the name and title section, with added entries taking the form of cross-references to the main entry. Each citation includes standard bibliographic information and, when available, the LC card number and the International Standard Book Number (ISBN) or International Standard Serial Number (ISSN).

The NLM *Classification Scheme* (4th edition, 1978, revised 1981) was generally used, although titles in peripheral fields were classified according to the LC classification schedules with no modification. Subject headings are from *MeSH (Medical Subject Headings)*, NLM's controlled vocabulary list, which is also used in the preparation of the other NLM bibliographies and indexes. Individuals and corporate bodies appearing as subjects are listed in the name and title section rather than in the subject section.

From 1973 through 1983 cataloged reference materials were brought together under the heading "REFERENCE BOOKS, MEDICAL" in the subject section for monographs. They are listed in a separate section, "Medical Reference Works," from 1984 through 1993.

    2.3 *Online Computer Library Center (OCLC)*. Dublin, OH, Online Computer Library Center.
    2.4 *Research Libraries Information Network (RLIN)*. Mountain View, CA, Research Libraries Group.

OCLC and RLIN are national networking systems that provide cataloging records and bibliographic descriptions for a variety of materials, including monographs, in all subject areas. In addition to NLM, sources of cataloging information include member libraries, Library of Congress MARC tapes, and the British Library.

    Each database contains millions of records and is updated continuously, throughout the day. These systems are major sources of bibliographic information on monographs. They are also important sources of location information, because each system indicates the holding libraries for items in its database.

    Other general bibliographic tools, such as the *National Union Catalog (NUC), Cumulative Book Index, American Book Publishing Record,* and *Weekly Record*, are also useful in the verification and location of medical monographs. However, these sources are likely to be available only in the largest health sciences libraries.

    2.5 *National Union Catalog*. Washington, DC, Library of Congress, 1983- . Monthly. Microfiche. Continues: *National Union Catalog: A Cumulative Author List*. Washington, DC, Library of Congress, 1956-1982.
    2.6 *Cumulative Book Index*. New York, H. W. Wilson, 1898- . Monthly (except August), annual cumulation.
    2.7 *American Book Publishing Record*. New Providence, NJ, R. R. Bowker, 1961- . Monthly; annual cumulation.
    2.8 *Weekly Record*. New Providence, NJ, R. R. Bowker, 1974- . Weekly.

The *National Union Catalog* provides a listing of materials currently cataloged by LC, regardless of imprint date, and by participating libraries throughout the United States and Canada, for imprints 1956 and later, if the material has not previously been cataloged by LC. Because of the extremely large number of items included in *NUC*, it represents a vast bibliographic resource for a large part of the world's output of monographs and other types of material.

    The series of catalogs published by NLM from 1948 to 1965 served as supplements to the LC catalogs in the field of medicine and related subjects.

With the inauguration of the *Current Catalog* in 1966, the NLM catalog was no longer a supplement to the LC catalogs. Catalog entries from NLM with an imprint date of 1956 or later are included in the *NUC*, as are entries for works in medicine acquired and cataloged by the Library of Congress and by the other participating libraries. For an extensive discussion of the history, development, and scope of the *NUC*, the reader is referred to the foreword that appeared in each issue of the printed version.

The microfiche *National Union Catalog* is published in a register/index format in four parts: NUC Books, NUC U.S. Books, NUC AV, and NUC Cartographic Materials. Each of these parts appears as a register with four indexes: name, title, subject, and series. Items in the register are numbered in sequence as they are added, and these records include all the elements traditionally found on LC printed cards. Items in the indexes are shortened versions of the full register record and are in alphabetical order.

Entries may appear in the *NUC* only if a participating library has acquired and cataloged an item; thus *NUC* serves not only as a verification source but also as a location source.

Monographs listed in *NUC* with a publication date of 1968 or later can be searched on CD-ROM and online through DIALOG, WILSONLINE, OCLC, and RLIN.

The *Cumulative Book Index (CBI)* and the *American Book Publishing Record* represent two continuing sources that attempt to provide bibliographic information about English-language publications in all subject areas. As such, they are important to health sciences librarians. Their primary purpose is to list books that can be purchased from publishers, and each provides enough information to order an item. Over a period of time, their cumulations provide a record of English-language monographs published in the United States or elsewhere.

The *American Book Publishing Record* and its companion work, the *Weekly Record*, provide a monthly and weekly listing of new books published only in the United States. The *Cumulative Book Index* has a broader scope: Its goal is to provide an international bibliography of books in the English language. *CBI* is also available online through WILSONLINE and on CD-ROM.

    2.9 *Books in Print*. New Providence, NJ, R. R. Bowker, 1948- . Annual.
    Books in Print Supplement. New Providence, NJ, R. R. Bowker, 1973- . Annual.
    2.10 *Medical and Health Care Books and Serials in Print*. New Providence, NJ, R. R. Bowker, 1985- , 2 vols. Continues: *Medical Books and Serials in Print*, 1978-1984.
    2.11 *Canadian Books in Print*. Toronto, University of Toronto Press, 1973- . Annual, with microfiche supplement.

A recurring question in bibliographic work involves the availability for purchase of a particular item: Is it still in print and for sale? The following publications offer assistance with this type of question.

Books in Print (BIP) covers all subject areas and provides an author and title approach to more than 1.2 million books that are still in print. Each entry includes the source from which the book can be purchased and its cost, along with other bibliographic elements, such as year of publication, ISBN, and LC card number. The addresses for publishers included in *BIP* are listed in a separate volume. Most of the titles listed in *BIP* can be found in the *Subject Guide to Books in Print*, which uses LC subject headings. *Books in Print* is available online through BRS and DIALOG, and on CD-ROM and microfiche as BIP Plus.

BIP and the *Subject Guide* are prepared from a computer database maintained by R.R. Bowker to compile its various in-print publications. Another reference source produced from this database is *Medical and Health Care Books and Serials in Print*—a title of direct interest to health sciences librarians. This work is a cumulation of more than 65,000 titles in the health sciences and allied fields. It contains monographs that are in print and have been or will be published or exclusively distributed in the United States. This source is likely to be of greatest value to the smaller library that cannot afford to have an extensive collection of bibliographic tools. It can be searched on the BIP Plus and the SciTech Reference Plus CD-ROMs.

Canadian Books in Print (CBIP) is intended primarily to bridge the gap between *Books in Print* and *British Books in Print*. Listings in *CBIP* are based on information supplied by Canadian publishers. The *Author and Title Index* is issued quarterly—a hardcover annual edition with complete microfiche editions in April, July, and October. The *Subject Index* is published annually in hardcover only. *CBIP* is available online through Info Globe Online.

RETROSPECTIVE SOURCES

The printed book was the primary source of information from the development of the printing press in the 15th century until the mid-19th century, by which time the periodical had so increased in use and number that it replaced the book in importance. Larger amounts of materials were being printed, and the sheer bulk of the literature made it impossible to be aware of everything being published.

Bibliographies of medical materials had been published prior to the mid-19th century, but they were selective in their coverage and had not attempted to be all-inclusive. They were concerned primarily with books, although the contents of periodicals were included in some bibliographies. In the early periods, many medical items were included in the general bibliographic tools and in those that were concerned solely or primarily with medical materials. For a detailed account of early bibliographic coverage of medical materials, the reader should consult *The Development of Medical Bibliography*, by Estelle Brodman [2]; for coverage since World War II, consult *Medical Bibliography in an Age of Discontinuity*, by Scott Adams [3].

The "father of medical bibliography" was John Shaw Billings, librarian of the Surgeon-General's Library, the forerunner of NLM. Billings was responsible for publication of the *Index Catalogue of the Library of the Surgeon-General's Office* and for the original *Index Medicus (IM)*. These publications marked the beginning of a consistent and systematized attempt to provide continuing bibliographic coverage of medical materials from all countries.

> 2.12 *Index Catalogue of the Library of the Surgeon-General's Office*. Ser. 1-5. Washington, DC, U.S. Government Printing Office, 1880-1961, 61 vols.
> 2.13 *Index Medicus: A Monthly Classified Record of the Current Medical Literature of the World*. Ser. 1-3. Various publishers, 1879-1927, 45 vols.

The *Index Catalogue*, first published in 1880, included all the monographic and periodical literature received by what was then the Library of the Surgeon-General's Office, and which became successively the Army Medical Library, the Armed Forces Medical Library, and the National Library of Medicine.

The *Index Catalogue* appeared in five series from 1880 to 1961, each of which contained a single alphabet, with author and subject entries appearing in dictionary form. Entries for monographs were listed under both the authors' names and subject headings; periodical articles were entered only under subject headings. Items were included in the *Index Catalogue* as they were acquired by the library; thus, many older items may be found in later series of the work. More than 500,000 monographs and 2.5 million journal articles are listed in these series. (Journal articles were dropped in later series.)

It must be remembered that the set is the catalog of one library and as such is a record of that library's holdings. The *Index Catalogue* is not a complete medical bibliography. However, the comprehensiveness of this collection that eventually became the National Library of Medicine makes the catalog the most extensive record available of the medical literature of the period.

In its time, the importance of the *Index Catalogue* was great. Today it is considered a valuable retrospective bibliography to have in any large medical or university library. It is a valuable historical source because of the early works that have been included.

Because each successive series was being published over a period of many years, it was necessary to have some means of bringing the *Index Catalogue* up to date. For this purpose, Billings created the *Index Medicus*, which was published from 1879 to 1927 with several breaks. It contained entries for books and journal articles and included many entries not found elsewhere. Its arrangement was by subject with an author index. *IM* was initially published monthly and then quarterly.

2.14 National Library of Medicine. *Catalog, 1948-1965.* Washington, DC, Library of Congress, annual; five-year cumulations, beginning 1950/1954-1965.

From 1948 until 1965, these volumes were published as a supplement to the printed catalogs issued by LC. They also serve as a bridge for monographs between the final series of the *Index Catalogue*, which covered monographs published up to 1950, and the *National Library of Medicine Current Catalog*, the printed catalog derived from the CATLINE database. Each volume includes cataloging information for monographs cataloged during the period, regardless of the monograph's date of publication.

2.15 *National Union Catalog: Pre-1956 Imprints.* London, Mansell, 1968-1980, 685 vols. *Supplement,* 1980-1981, vols. 686-754.

The Library of Congress' cumulative publication of its printed catalogs prior to 1956, plus previously unpublished material located in the *National Union Catalog,* represents another significant source of information for older monographs and serial titles in the health sciences. *Pre-1956 Imprints* contains, in one alphabetical listing, entries for materials published prior to January 1, 1956, that have been cataloged by the LC or by one of the participating libraries in the NUC. It comprises one of the largest sets of printed materials in the world.

2.16 *The American Book Publishing Record Cumulative: 1876-1949.* New York, R. R. Bowker, 1980, 15 vols. *The American Book Publishing Record Cumulative: 1950-1977,* 1979, 15 vols.
2.17 *Health Science Books 1876-1982.* New York, R. R. Bowker, 1982.

Virtually every book in every field published and distributed in the United States between 1876 and 1977 is included in the two *American Book Publishing Record Cumulatives.* More than 1.5 million titles, with full bibliographic and cataloging information on each, have been taken from the *American Book Publishing Record* database, the *National Union Catalog,* and the Library of Congress MARC tapes.

Health Science Books 1876-1982 represents more than 133,000 titles—in all areas of the health sciences—published or distributed in the United States and cataloged by the Library of Congress between 1876 and 1982.

REFERENCES

1. Katz WA. Introduction to reference work. Volume one: Basic information sources. 6th ed. New York: McGraw-Hill, 1992:61.

2. Brodman E. The development of medical bibliography. Baltimore: Medical Library Association, 1954.

3. Adams S. Medical bibliography in an age of discontinuity. Chicago: Medical Library Association, 1981.

READINGS

Adams S. Medical bibliography in an age of discontinuity. Chicago: Medical Library Association, 1981.

Brodman E. The development of medical bibliography. Baltimore: Medical Library Association, 1954.

Grogan D. Bibliographies. In: Science and technology: An introduction to the literature. 4th ed. rev., London: Clive Bingley, 1982:117-30.

Katz WA. Bibliographies: National library catalogs and trade bibliographies. In: Introduction to reference work. Volume one: Basic information sources. 6th ed. New York: McGraw-Hill, 1992:89-118.

Sutherland FM. Use of medical literature. 2d ed. London: Butterworths, 1977:39-61.

CHAPTER 3

Bibliographic Sources for Periodicals

Fred W. Roper

The periodicals collection constitutes the major element of most health sciences libraries' holdings. Thus, there is a strong need for tools that assist in the identification and verification of periodical titles. Because no single library can ever acquire enough materials to be self-sufficient, bibliographic sources that give locations for periodicals are essential. In addition, the health sciences librarian is continually concerned with collection development and the selection of titles to be added to or dropped from the library's holdings.

To perform these various functions, the reference collection must contain a variety of bibliographic sources—both those that specialize in the health sciences and those of a more general nature—that deal primarily or in part with periodicals. Included among these sources are bibliographies of periodicals, online databases, and union catalogs.

HISTORICAL NOTE

It was not until 1665 that the scientific periodical as a publishing form came into existence. The *Journal des Scavans*, first published on January 5, 1665, is considered the first learned journal. Soon after the initial appearance of the *Journal*, the Royal Society (London) began publication of the *Philosophical Transactions of the Royal Society*. The *Journal* was aimed at the amateur, while *Philosophical Transactions* was intended to serve as a "means of communication between practising scientists, as well as a journal of interesting and curious knowledge" [1].

Since these beginnings in the 17th century, the number of scientific periodicals has increased at an extremely rapid rate, particularly since the mid-20th century. The periodical is now the vehicle for first publication of research results and for timely communication with colleagues. The book, on the other hand, has been relegated the task of "the formal and proper publication of mature reflections or a completed opus..." rather than the reporting of work currently in progress [2].

CURRENT SOURCES

Bibliographic work with periodicals can be a challenge to the librarian because of the many vagaries associated with them. Changes are constantly taking place—title variations, new publishing pattern and format, cessations, and rebirths are just a few of the possibilities.

The sheer number of periodical publications makes it difficult for the librarian to be aware of what has been and is being published. The large number of titles stems partly from the "publish-or-perish" syndrome and partly from spin-offs of periodicals, which create new and separate titles. A related problem occurs when authors submit either the same article or reworked material to more than one publication.

A variety of sources provide information about the status of currently published periodicals. The National Library of Medicine's SERLINE and CATLINE systems and their byproducts are of primary importance to health sciences librarians.

3.1 *SERLINE (SERials onLINE)*. Bethesda, MD, National Library of Medicine.

3.2 *Health Sciences Serials*. Bethesda, MD, National Library of Medicine, 1978- . Quarterly. Microfiche.

3.3 *CATLINE (CATalog onLINE)*. Bethesda, MD, National Library of Medicine.

3.4 *National Library of Medicine Current Catalog*. Bethesda, MD, National Library of Medicine, 1966-1993. Annual cumulations.

3.5 *List of Serials Indexed for Online Users*. Bethesda, MD, National Library of Medicine, 1980- . Annual.

SERLINE contains bibliographic citations for all serials and numbered congresses on order, in process, or cataloged for the NLM collection, as well as a limited number of serials that are selectively indexed by NLM but not held in the collection. Periodical titles held by libraries participating in SERHOLD are also included in SERLINE. Information such as title changes and ceased titles is provided as well. There are more than 80,000 titles in the database and about 140 new records are added with each monthly update. The addition of location symbols for approximately 150 resource libraries in the National Network of Libraries of Medicine (NN/LM) permits SERLINE to serve as both a bibliographic record and a source of location information for interlibrary loan work.

Health Sciences Serials, a SERLINE product, is a quarterly publication distributed in microfiche that contains the same information as the SER-LINE database. In addition, location information is included for approximately 120 other medical libraries in the NN/LM.

In Chapter 2, CATLINE was described as a source of information for monographs and serials that have been cataloged or recataloged at NLM since 1965. Although the CATLINE and SERLINE files do overlap, CAT-LINE contains some serials not found in SERLINE. In addition, the bibliographic elements in CATLINE represent full cataloging information.

The *National Library of Medicine Current Catalog* contains cataloging data arranged by main entry and by subject for NLM serials cataloged from 1965 through 1993.

The *List of Serials Indexed for Online Users* is designed to provide complete bibliographic information on serials cited in four MEDLARS (MEDical Literature Analysis and Retrieval System) files: MEDLINE (MEDlars on-LINE), including the BACKFILES; HEALTH (HEALTH planning and administration); POPLINE (POPulation information onLINE); and BIOTECHSEEK (BIOSEEK). Selected citations from those files are published in bibliographies such as *Index Medicus (IM), Index to Dental Literature, International Nursing Index,* and *Hospital Literature Index.*

List of Serials contains ceased titles, changed titles, titles no longer indexed, and titles currently indexed. It is an alphabetical list of title abbreviations (no full-title list is provided) for more than 8,000 publications, of which 3,738 titles are presently indexed by NLM. Elements of information include the city of publication, first/last indicator, journal title code, indexing status, the ISSN, NLM call number, and NLM title control number, which is used by medical libraries in reporting serial holdings data to SERHOLD.

Most of the serials currently indexed appear in *Index Medicus.* If the serial is not an *IM* title, a symbol indicates the index (e.g., *Index to Dental Literature*) or database (e.g., POPLINE) for which the title is indexed. *List of Serials* serves as a bridge between the online databases and the available printed tools.

3.6 *Medical and Health Care Books and Serials in Print.* New Providence, NJ, R. R. Bowker, 1985- . 2 vols. Continues: *Medical Books and Serials in Print,* 1978-1984.

Medical and Health Care Books and Serials in Print provides international coverage of "selected titles of periodicals issued more frequently than once a year and usually published at regular intervals, and/or irregular serials and annuals provided the last issue date was not earlier than 1968" (Preface). The 15,000 entries for serials have been taken from the same database used to compile Bowker's *Ulrich's International Periodicals Directory*. The serials listed in *Medical and Health Care Books* and *Serials in Print* can also be searched on CD-ROM as a part of Ulrich's Plus and SciTech Reference Plus.

> 3.7 *Ulrich's International Periodicals Directory*. New Providence, NJ, R. R. Bowker, 1932- . Annual. Absorbed: *Irregular Serials and Annuals*, 1967-1987/1988.
>
> 3.8 *Ulrich's Update*. New Providence, NJ, R. R. Bowker, 1988- . Continues: *Bowker International Serials Database Update*, 1985-1988, *Ulrich's Quarterly*, 1977-1985.
>
> 3.9 *The Serials Directory: An International Reference Book*. Birmingham, AL, EBSCO, 1986- . Annual. 3 vols.

These publications will be useful because of the wide range of titles beyond the health sciences likely to be included in a library's periodicals collection.

Ulrich's International Periodicals Directory provides information on nearly 140,000 titles currently being published throughout the world. It includes serials published more frequently than once a year and publications issued annually or less frequently than once a year, or irregularly. More than 6,500 refereed serials are listed. *Ulrich's Update*, published three times a year, includes new serial titles, a title change index, and a listing of cessations. The *Ulrich's* database can be searched on CD-ROM, microfiche, and online through DIALOG and BRS.

The Serials Directory has more than 155,000 titles of international serials, annuals, and irregular serials. There is a ceased titles index that lists 11,000 serials. The peer reviewed/refereed index includes current and ceased serials that contain peer-reviewed articles. Cumulative updates are published throughout the year. The CD-ROM version of *The Serials Directory* provides access to more than 180,000 titles.

Lists from Indexing and Abstracting Services

The major indexing and abstracting services in the health sciences provide lists of the periodicals they index and abstract on a regular basis. These lists serve as important supplements to the more inclusive bibliographies of current periodicals.

> 3.10 *List of Journals Indexed in Index Medicus*. Bethesda, MD, National Library of Medicine, 1960- . Annual.
>
> 3.11 Excerpta Medica. *List of Journals Indexed*. Amsterdam, Excerpta Medica, 1964- . Annual. Continues: *List of Journals Abstracted*.

3.12 *Serial Sources for the BIOSIS Previews Database.* Philadelphia, PA, BioSciences Information Service, 1978- . Annual. Continues: *Serial Sources for the BIOSIS Data Base.*

3.13 *Science Citation Index Guide and Lists of Source Publications.* Philadelphia, PA, Institute for Scientific Information Service, 1977- . Annual.

3.14 *Chemical Abstracts Service Source Index, 1907-1989 Cumulative.* Columbus, OH, Chemical Abstract Service. 1980- . 3 vols. Quarterly supplements with annual cumulations.

The National Library of Medicine has selected more than 3,058 of the most important biomedical and health sciences journals for indexing in *IM*. The *List of Journals Indexed in Index Medicus (LJI)* arranges those titles in four sections: abbreviated title, full title, subject heading, and country of publication. Information provided in the abbreviated title section includes city of publication, the ISSN, NLM call number, and NLM title control number. Lists of title additions, deletions, and changes are also provided. *LJI* is kept up to date in the monthly NLM *Technical Bulletin* and in the July issue of *Index Medicus*.

Excerpta Medica's *List of Journals Indexed* is an annual publication of more than 3,500 serial titles. They are listed in three sections: abbreviated title, broad topic, and country of origin. The abbreviated title section gives the full title and publisher (including address and phone number) and also indicates if the journal is indexed cover-to-cover or selectively.

Serial Sources for the BIOSIS Previews Database contains entries for more than 18,900 titles—those presently being covered in the BIOSIS products and archival entries no longer being actively covered. Additional sections include information on changes that have taken place for individual titles.

The *Guide and Lists of Source Publications* provides information on the serial titles covered by *Science Citation Index (SCI)*. Lists of publications are arranged by title abbreviation, full title with publisher, new titles, subject, and country of origin. This source also serves as an introductory textbook for teaching uses of *SCI*.

The *Chemical Abstracts Service Source Index (CASSI)* includes information on titles included in the various CAS sources and provides a variety of other types of information. The *Chemical Abstracts Service Source Index, 1907-1989 Cumulative* includes all 120,099 entries published in *CASSI* through 1989. It is updated on a quarterly basis and provides complete bibliographic information. *CASSI* also functions as a union list because it gives location information for the CAS titles in major libraries. Online access is provided through ORBIT.

Periodicals Holdings Information

Sources that reveal library holdings of periodicals are essential in locating the nearest centers for borrowing or for photocopying desired articles. Although printed union lists continue to be useful for identifying libraries that hold a particular item, online systems are usually the first sources consulted when searching for this information.

> 3.15 *DOCLINE*. Bethesda, MD, National Library of Medicine.

DOCLINE is NLM's online interlibrary loan (ILL) request and referral system for health sciences libraries. Because DOCLINE is linked to SERLINE and other NLM databases, the borrowing library enters the unique citation number included in those records and the system automatically places all the necessary bibliographic data in the ILL request. The request is then routed throughout the NN/LM, which comprises more than 3,400 health sciences libraries and information centers.

A major component of DOCLINE is the automatic routing of requests for titles in SERHOLD, NLM's database of holdings statements for serial titles held by U.S. health sciences libraries. SERHOLD is also the source of location information that appears in SERLINE and *Health Sciences Serials* and is used to produce a variety of union lists.

OCLC, RLIN, and the Western Library Network (WLN) are also primary sources for holdings information and each provides ILL service to libraries.

In addition to these online sources, the librarian must remember to use the other sources that are available when searching for locations of holding libraries.

Libraries publish individual lists, with variations as to the intent of each list and the amount of information offered. These lists will range from current subscription lists to catalogs of all titles held by the library, ceased and current, with complete holdings information. Union lists range from national lists to regional and local union catalogs that reveal holdings within an area. As aids to bibliographic verification and location, they are indispensable in a reference collection, and the reference librarian needs to be aware of union lists that can be of immediate assistance.

> 3.16 *UCMP Quarterly*. New York, Medical Library Center of New York, 1973- . Quarterly. Microfiche.

A good example of a regional health sciences periodicals holdings list is *UCMP Quarterly*. This union catalog represents the holdings of 770 libraries in Delaware, New Jersey, New York, Pennsylvania, and the New England region. Included are approximately 75,000 periodical titles; in addition to holdings information, there are bibliographic notes giving the history of each title with dates and frequency of publication. Each issue revises and cumulates previous issues. *UCMP Quarterly* is the official union list for regions 1 and 8 of the NN/LM. The *Quarterly* plans to go online by early 1995.

3.17 *New Serial Titles.* Washington, DC, Library of Congress, 1953- . Eight issues per year; quarterly and annual cumulations.

3.18 *New Serial Titles: A Union List of Serials Commencing Publication After December 31, 1949; 1950-1970 Subject Guide.* New York, R. R. Bowker, 1975. 2 vols.

3.19 *Union List of Serials in Libraries of the United States and Canada.* 3d ed. New York, H. W. Wilson, 1965. 5 vols.

3.20 *World List of Scientific Periodicals Published in the Years 1900-1960.* 4th ed. Washington, DC, Butterworths, 1963.

3.21 *British Union-Catalogue of Periodicals.* New York, Academic Press, 1955. *Supplement to 1960.* Washington, DC, Butterworths, 1962.

3.22 *Serials in the British Library.* London, British Library, 1981- . Quarterly, annual cumulation. Continues: *British Union-Catalogue of Periodicals: New Periodical Titles,* 1964-1980.

New Serial Titles, produced by the Library of Congress (LC), reflects the titles reported by LC or by one of the participating libraries in the *National Union Catalog.* It is intended to provide bibliographic and holdings information of serials that have begun publication since 1950, and as such it serves as a supplement to the *Union List of Serials.* It appears in eight monthly issues with three quarterly issues cumulating the two previous months and including the current one. These issues in turn appear as an annual cumulation. Annual editions are cumulated every five years. (A twenty-year cumulation, *New Serial Titles, 1950-1970,* was published in 1973.) As libraries continue to report a title, new locations are listed in each succeeding cumulation. For titles that began publication prior to 1950, the *Union List of Serials* must be consulted.

These two titles give extensive coverage to periodicals from all countries, in all languages, and in all subject areas as long as the periodicals are held by a library in the United States or Canada that reports its holdings.

In Great Britain, two titles of importance are the *World List of Scientific Periodicals* and the *British Union-Catalogue of Periodicals.* The fourth edition of the *World List,* which appeared from 1963 to 1965, covers scientific, technical, and medical periodicals published from 1900 to 1960 that are held in British libraries. The *British Union-Catalogue of Periodicals* and its supplement cover periodicals from the 17th century to 1960, from all over the world and in all subject areas, as long as they are held in reporting British libraries.

New Periodical Titles united the *British Union-Catalogue of Periodicals* with the *World List of Scientific Periodicals*. It cumulated annually into two volumes. One volume covered all titles included in the quarterly issues and the other included only the scientific, technical, and medical entries. *New Periodical Titles* is continued by *Serials in the British Library*, which appears in three quarterly issues with the fourth issue being a one-volume annual cumulation. The majority of periodicals are listed by full title; when applicable, the entry provides title change information. The microfiche version of *Serials in the British Library* is issued annually and cumulates the listings in the quarterly printed publication.

Another important union list in the sciences is the *Chemical Abstracts Service Source Index*, which identifies the holding libraries of periodicals indexed by the Chemical Abstracts Service. The *CASSI, 1907-1979 Cumulative* also included location information for titles indexed by Engineering Index, the Institute for Scientific Information, and the BioSciences Information Service of Biological Abstracts (BIOSIS).

ABBREVIATIONS

The reference librarian is often asked to help in the identification of serial titles' abbreviations, which are usually from a bibliography in a monograph or periodical article. The major problem associated with this type of request is the lack of standardization that is observed in the formulation of abbreviations. Although standards have been developed by the American National Standards Institute (Z39 Subcommittee on Periodical Title Abbreviations), actual practice continues to vary.

Lack of regard for standardization has led to similar abbreviations for different titles and to varied abbreviations for the same title. All of the major indexing and abstracting services include an approach by abbreviated periodical title in their lists of titles indexed. In addition to these titles, *World List of Scientific Periodicals* and the *British Union-Catalogue of Periodicals* also offer access by abbreviation.

When the same abbreviation is used for multiple titles, further detective work is required to determine which title is needed. The publishing history of the titles will have to be examined, and a source that provides complete bibliographic information will need to be consulted. SERLINE, *Ulrich's International Periodicals Directory, Chemical Abstracts Service Source Index, UCMP Quarterly, New Serial Titles, Union List of Serials, World List of Scientific Periodicals,* and *British Union-Catalogue of Periodicals* will be of particular value when verifying an abbreviated title.

CHANGES

Another challenge of periodicals work is keeping up with the changes that take place in the bibliographic record of a periodical. The most common changes are new periodicals (births), cessations (deaths), and title changes. Obviously any element in the bibliographic record may change, but these are the major problem areas.

Sources that have special sections to note changes in periodical information include *Ulrich's International Periodicals Directory*, *Ulrich's Update*, *The Serials Directory*, *List of Journals Indexed in Index Medicus*, *Serial Sources for the BIOSIS Previews Database*, *Chemical Abstracts Service Source Index*, *New Serial Titles*, and *New Periodical Titles*.

REFERENCES

1. Brodman E. The development of medical bibliography. Baltimore: Medical Library Association, 1954:49-50.

2. Grogan D. Science and technology: an introduction to the literature. 4th ed, rev. London: Clive Bingley, 1982:131.

READINGS

Grogan D. Periodicals. In: Science and technology: an introduction to the literature. 4th ed. London: Clive Bingley, 1982:131-83.

Houghton B. Scientific periodicals: their historical development, characteristics and control. London: Clive Bingley, 1975.

International Committee of Medical Journal Editors. Uniform requirements for manuscripts submitted to biomedical journals. BMJ 1991 302:338-41.

Katz WA. Bibliographies: national library catalogs and trade bibliographies. In: Introduction to reference work. Volume one: Basic information sources. 6th ed. New York: McGraw-Hill, 1992:118-26.

Kronick DA. A history of scientific and technical periodicals: the origins and development of the scientific and technical press, 1665-1790. 2d ed. Metuchen, NJ: Scarecrow, 1976.

CHAPTER 4

Indexing and Abstracting Services

Jo Anne Boorkman

Indexing and abstracting services are designed to provide access to periodical and other literature through a variety of approaches. Subjects, in the form of either keywords or thesaurus terms, are frequently used as access points; however, approaches by authors and cited authors (authors listed in the bibliography of an article or book) are also possible. An index provides the basic bibliographic information needed to locate an article: name of author(s), article title, journal title, journal volume and year, and pages of the article. An abstracting service provides the same information but in addition includes a brief summary of an article's content—an abstract.

Indexing and abstracting services vary widely in the way they provide access to the bibliographic information that they are presenting. It is, therefore, important to evaluate the services by criteria that will give an idea of their value and their ease of use.

In using these services to help requesters develop bibliographies, verify references, and find information, it is essential to know the scope and coverage of each service. Not only is subject coverage important to note, but also the depth of coverage and types of materials indexed—journals, books, dissertations, government documents, etc. If a journal is indexed, are all the articles included, or just selected ones? Are brief reports indexed? Are substantive letters to the editor indexed? The number of serials indexed should also be noted, as well as languages and time period covered.

The number and types of indexes can vary with the scope and type of material covered by a service. Subject and author indexes are generally found in all, while report number, patent, molecular formula, systematic, and citation indexes are found in specialized indexing and abstracting services. Some author indexes list only the first author of a paper, while others include additional authors. It is important to know the policy of an index as to whether all an author's writings will be listed or just the ones for which he or she is the primary author.

Subject indexes take all sorts of forms. Some subject indexes are strictly keyword indexes created by extracting terms from the title of an article, while others augment the keywords from titles with additional terms provided by indexers. In still other instances, the indexes use a controlled vocabulary or thesaurus, where subject descriptors are assigned by indexers to describe the content of the article referenced. Whether a strictly defined term must be used to look up references on a subject (e.g., MeSH descriptors with *Index Medicus*) or a variety of synonyms are provided to cover that subject (e.g., the *Permuterm Subject Index* of *Science Citation Index*) will make a big difference in the analysis of a bibliographic question. The choice of initial index is often based on how easily the subject can be searched when one uses the structure of the subject index.

Two types of keyword indexes that should be mentioned are the Keyword in Context (KWIC) and the Keyword Out of Context (KWOC). A KWIC index takes keywords as they appear in the title of an article and lists the title in the index alphabetically under each significant word. An augmented KWIC index would include terms selected from the abstract by an indexer. An example of this type of index is that used by the BioSciences Information Service (BIOSIS) in the subject index to *Biological Abstracts*. The KWOC index employs all significant words from the title and does not list them with the title, but instead refers to the complete citation by reference number or author's name. For example, a listing from the *Permuterm Subject Index* of *Science Citation Index* would look like this:

Chain-reaction
   detection   — Atmar RL
                  — Biswas J
   evaluation   — Thiele D
                  — Wang JT

In some services the indexes are very brief in the monthly or quarterly issues, listing citations by broad subject classification and limiting detailed indexes to semiannual or annual cumulations.

The arrangement of the information can vary widely in both indexes and abstracts. The sequence of bibliographic elements for an entry as well as where the unit entry (the entry where the complete bibliographic reference is given) is listed should be noted. The most commonly used formats list unit entries in a classified, author, subject, or journal title arrangement. Generally, the indexes arrange references directly under author or subject or both, as in *Index Medicus*. Abstracting services, as a rule, arrange the references with abstracts in classified or broad subject arrangement with author, detailed subject, and special indexes referring to the citation or reference number in the classified section. *Excerpta Medica* and *Biological Abstracts* both follow this format. If foreign-language articles are indexed, the language in which the title appears should be noted. For translated titles, the language of the article should be indicated. The availability of an English abstract in the journal is also noteworthy in an index. For further assessment of an abstracting service, the source of an abstract—signed, anonymous, or from the journal—can indicate whether the abstract is critical or simply a summary of the article. Generally, signed abstracts are written by subject specialists and are more critical than author abstracts.

Publication characteristics of the service should also be considered. What is the average time between the publication of an original article and its appearance in an indexing or abstracting journal? The frequency of publication of the indexing or abstracting service has some bearing on the time lag associated with a reference's appearance. However, abstracting services tend to have a longer time lag than indexing services.

The value of any indexing or abstracting service will also depend on how easy it is to use. However, even complicated formats can be helpful, provided the service gives information on how best to use its product. Therefore, further criteria to look for are whether the service has provided a guide to using the indexing or abstracting source, a list of journals, other material covered by the service, and a list of journal title abbreviations.

Another factor to consider is the cost of the service, not just in relation to the library's budget but also in relation to the other indexing and abstracting services in a library's collection. In this context, uniqueness of coverage should be weighed against overlap of coverage. The service's usefulness as a reference tool in terms of the needs of the library's primary clientele must be considered as well.

In the following review of the major indexing and abstracting services in the health sciences, the criteria discussed above will be used: coverage, access to information, arrangement of information, and publication characteristics. Some libraries will undoubtedly also have to weigh the usefulness of these tools to their clientele against budgetary constraints. The printed versions of these services are discussed in this chapter. The online databases and their capabilities will be discussed in the next chapter.

INDEX MEDICUS

4.1 *Index Medicus*. Bethesda, MD, National Library of Medicine. Monthly. Vol. 1- , 1960- .

The *Index Medicus(IM)* is the major index to medical periodical literature. The *Index Medicus* (New Series) began in 1960. Its predecessors—beginning with the *Index Catalogue of the Library of the Surgeon General's Office*, volume 1, 1880, and the *Index Medicus*, volume 1, 1879, and followed by the *Quarterly Cumulative Index to Current Medical Literature*—will not be discussed here (*see* Figure 4-1). A brief history of these publications and their relationship to one another is in the introduction to *Cumulated Index Medicus*, volume 1, 1960 [1-2].

Index Medicus appears monthly and cumulates annually. The first five cumulative volumes (volumes 1-5, 1960-1964) were published by the American Medical Association (AMA) with subsequent cumulative volumes published by the National Library of Medicine (NLM). The current index is broad in coverage, indexing 3,058 journals in the medical and health-related sciences. Selected monographs and conference proceedings from the international literature were included from May 1976-1982. Approximately half the citations refer to articles in languages other than English, indicated by brackets around the English translation of the title, with the original language noted at the end of the citation. In the early 1960s, NLM began developing its computerized bibliographic database, the *MEDical Literature Analysis and Retrieval System* (MEDLARS), for producing *Index Medicus* [3-4]. Since 1966, the format of *Index Medicus* has remained essentially the same.

The bulk of the index has a subject arrangement with full references listed directly under each subject heading. Subject headings are assigned by indexers at NLM using a controlled vocabulary, *MeSH* (*Medical Subject Headings*). Subject headings are further delineated by the use of subheadings. For example, an article on the anatomy of the eye would be listed under "EYE"/anatomy and histology; an article on the use of penicillin to treat a disease would be found under "PENICILLIN"/therapeutic use. Indexers are instructed to assign the most specific subject headings or subject heading/subheading combinations to describe the *contents* of an article. Therefore, it is important to determine the appropriate subject headings for a topic by using *MeSH* before approaching *Index Medicus*. As a further example, an article on the physiology of the retina of the eye will be indexed under "RETINA"/physiology but *not* "EYE"/physiology because the article is on the retina, a specific part of the eye, and not the eye in general.

MeSH is revised annually, with new terms added and old terms either changed to current terminology or deleted. There are four published forms of *MeSH* to help select appropriate subject headings: an alphabetic list that appears annually as Part Two of the January issue of *Index Medicus*; an annotated alphabetic list (Figure 4-2); a tree structure (Figure 4-3), which is a hierarchical arrangement of the subject terms; and a permuted list (Figure 4-4).

Figure 4-1. Medical Indexes to Periodical Literature

Index Medicus J. S. Billings, et al.	1879-99; series I 1903-20; series II 1921-27; series III	Monthly publication Indexing periodical literature
Bibliographia Medica Paris, Institut de Bibliographic	1900-03, vols. 1-3	Covers the years between series I and series II of *Index Medicus*
Index Catalogue J. S. Billings, et al.	1880-95;1st series, 16 vols.	Indexing monographs and periodicals
	1896-16; 2nd series, 21 vols.	Indexing monographs and periodicals
	1918-32; 3rd series, 10 vols.	Indexing monographs and periodicals
	1936-48; 4th series, 11 vols. (A-MEZ)	Indexing monographs and periodicals
	1955; 4th series, 1 vol. (Mh-Mn)	
	1959, 1961; 5th series, 3 vols.	Monographs only 1959 Authors and titles only 1961 Subjects A-M; N-Z
Quarterly Cumulative Index (QCI), AMA	1916-26; 12 volumes	Clinical journals indexed with some books and government documents
Quarterly Cumulative Index Medicus (QCIM), AMA	1927-56	Supersedes *Index Medicus* and *QCI*. Army Medical Library furnished some citations until 1932
Current List of Medical Literature (CLML)	1941-59	Published privately by A. Seidell, later assisted by the Army Medical Library; in 1945 the Army Medical Library took over the publication
Index Medicus (New Series)	1960-	Took the place of *QCIM* and superseded *CLML*

The alphabetic *MeSH* and annotated alphabetic *MeSH* (*see* Figure 4-2) provide cross-references from terms that are not subject headings to MeSH terms, as well as to related MeSH terms that could be appropriate to a topic. The date the term entered the vocabulary and tree numbers indicating in which categories the term belongs are also provided in both forms of the alphabetic *MeSH*. Notes on the use of a term and allowable subheadings are included in the annotated *MeSH* for use by indexers, catalogers, and searchers.

The *MeSH* tree structure (*see* Figure 4-3) provides a subject categorization of the vocabulary in fifteen sections, e.g., A. Anatomy, C. Diseases, D. Drugs and Chemicals. Each section is further broken down for specificity. The tree structure is an important tool in helping to select terms that are not easily scanned in the alphabetic *MeSH*. It is an even more important tool for online computer searching of the MEDLARS database, MEDLINE.

The permuted *MeSH* (*see* Figure 4-4) alphabetically lists each significant word from a subject heading or cross-reference. Arranged alphabetically under each word are all the MeSH terms and cross-references used in the thesaurus. This enables anyone unfamiliar with the vocabulary to access it without prior knowledge of its terminology.

In addition to the uses of *MeSH* for indexing and manual searching of *Index Medicus* and computer searching of MEDLINE, the MeSH vocabulary is used for cataloging and manual searching of NLM's *Current Catalog* and *Audiovisuals Catalog*, as well as computer searching of their online counterparts, CATLINE and AVLINE. It is further used by most health sciences libraries for subject cataloging of their collections for the public catalog.

Articles are indexed with twelve to sixteen subject headings but will be listed in the printed *Index Medicus* under three to five headings. English-language articles are listed first (alphabetically arranged by journal title abbreviation), and each entry includes the title, author, journal title, volume, page, and, for review articles, the number of references in the bibliography. Within each subheading category, foreign-language references follow those in English, with the language indicated in parentheses following the reference. The availability of an English abstract in the journal is also noted. The author index provides the bibliographic reference after the first author's name, with cross-references from additional authors' names referring to the first author. The author index also lists foreign-language titles in the language of publication.

A special feature of *IM* is the *Bibliography of Medical Reviews (BMR)* found in each monthly *IM* and cumulated in the annual. It has the same format as the main index but provides separate access by subject to lengthy and review articles. "Types of articles now considered to be reviews include academic, classical, or exhaustive reviews; tutorial, didactic or subject reviews; multicase or epidemiologic reviews; consensus conferences; re-

Figure 4-2. Annotated Alphabetic and Alphabetic *MeSH*

Annotated Alphabetic *MeSH*

QUALITY ASSURANCE, HEALTH CARE
N4.761.700+   N5.700+
DF: QUAL ASSUR   CATALOG: /geog /form
80; QUALITY ASSURANCE PROGRAM was see QUALITY OF HEALTH
CARE 1978–79
use QUALITY OF HEALTH CARE to search QUALITY ASSURANCE
PROGRAM 1978–79
X   QUALITY ASSESSMENT, HEALTH CARE

QUALITY CIRCLES see MANAGEMENT QUALITY CIRCLES
N4.452.677.420

QUALITY CONTROL
J1.897.608
NIM; no qualif
74(71)
see related
     REFERENCE STANDARDS

QUALITY OF HEALTH CARE
N4.761+   N5.715+
IM   CATALOG: /geog /form
68
see related
     NATIONAL PRACTITIONER DATA BANK
     PROFESSIONAL STAFF COMMITTEES

QUALITY OF LIFE
I1.800   K1.752.770
no qualif
77(75)
see related
     LIFE STYLE
XR COST OF ILLNESS
XR LIFE STYLE

QUANTUM THEORY
H1.671.579.800
67(64)

Alphabetic *MeSH*
(no annotations in this version)

QUALITY CIRCLES see MANAGEMENT QUALITY CIRCLES

QUALITY CONTROL
J1.897.608
74
see related
     REFERENCE STANDARDS

QUALITY OF HEALTH CARE
N4.761+   N5.715+
68
see related
     NATIONAL PRACTITIONER DATA BANK
     PROFESSIONAL STAFF COMMITTEES

QUALITY OF LIFE
I1.800   K1.752.770
77
see related
     LIFE STYLE
XR COST OF ILLNESS
XR LIFE STYLE

QUANTUM THEORY
H1.671.579.800
67

QUARANTINE
G3.850.780.200.450.700
see related
     PATIENT ISOLATION

QUARTZ
D1.836.751.636
91,63–64; was see under SILICA 1965–90; was heading 1963–64

Under QUALITY OF HEALTH CARE note:
   N4.761+ and N5.715+ --MeSH tree numbers, + indicates more specific terms are listed
   under these numbers
   IM--*Index Medicus* subject heading
   68--the date the term started being used in the MeSH vocabulary
   see related--other MeSH terms to consider

Under QUALITY OF LIFE note:
   no qualif--no subheadings are used with this term
   77(75)--77 is the date the term entered the vocabulary for use in *Index Medicus*; (75) the date
   indexers began using the term for online retrieval, listed in the Annotated *MeSH* only

National Library of Medicine, Medical subject headings, annotated alphabetic list, 1993 (Bethesda, MD:
National Library of Medicine, 1993), p. 798; Medical Subject Headings. *Index Medicus* 1993;
34(suppl):545.

Figure 4-3. *MeSH* Tree Structure

N4 – HEALTH CARE–HEALTH SERVICES ADMINISTRATION

HEALTH SERVICES ADMINISTRATION (NON MESH)
PATIENT CARE MANAGEMENT (NON MESH)
DELIVERY OF HEALTH CARE

DELIVERY OF HEALTH CARE	N4.590.374	N5.300	
HEALTH SERVICES ACCESSIBILITY	N4.590.374.200	N5.300.430	
MANAGED CARE PROGRAMS	N4.590.374.410	N3.219.521.	
COMPETITIVE MEDICAL PLANS	N4.590.374.410.175	N3.219.521.	
HEALTH MAINTENANCE ORGANIZATIONS	N4.590.374.410.400	N3.219.521. N4.452.758.	N3.219.521.
INDEPENDENT PRACTICE ASSOCIATIONS	N4.590.374.410.450	N3.219.521. N4.452.758.	N4.452.758.
PREFERRED PROVIDER ORGANIZATIONS	N4.590.374.410.750	N3.219.521.	
PRODUCT LINE MANAGEMENT	N4.590.374.600	N2.278.354.	N4.452.442.
TELEMEDICINE	N4.590.374.800	G2.403.840	L1.178.847.
PATIENT CARE TEAM	N4.590.715		
NURSING, TEAM	N4.590.715.571		
PHYSICIAN'S PRACTICE PATTERNS	N4.590.748	N5.300.625	
QUALITY OF HEALTH CARE	N4.761	N5.715	
MEDICAL AUDIT	N4.761.380	N5.700.500	
COMMISSION ON PROFESSIONAL AND HOSPITAL ACTIVITIES	N4.761.380.100	N5.700.500.	
NURSING AUDIT	N4.761.520	N5.700.520	
OUTCOME AND PROCESS ASSESSMENT (HEALTH CARE)	N4.761.559	N5.715.360.	
OUTCOME ASSESSMENT (HEALTH CARE)	N4.761.559.590	N5.715.360.	
TREATMENT OUTCOME	N4.761.559.590.800	E1.789.800	N5.715.360.
TREATMENT FAILURE	N4.761.559.590.800.760	E1.789.800.	N5.715.360.
PROCESS ASSESSMENT (HEALTH CARE)	N4.761.559.650	N5.715.360.	
PEER REVIEW	N4.761.610	L1.737.633	N5.700.600
PROFESSIONAL REVIEW ORGANIZATIONS	N4.761.673	N5.700.675	
PROGRAM EVALUATION	N4.761.685	E5.337.820	N5.715.360.
QUALITY ASSURANCE, HEALTH CARE	N4.761.700	N5.700	
GUIDELINES	N4.761.700.350	N5.700.350	
PRACTICE GUIDELINES	N4.761.700.350.650	N5.700.350.	
UTILIZATION REVIEW	N4.761.879	N5.700.900	
CONCURRENT REVIEW	N4.761.879.200	N5.700.900.	

N4.761--common tree number for QUALITY OF HEALTH CARE terms

N5.715--additional location of QUALITY OF HEALTH CARE in the tree

National Library of Medicine. Medical subject headings, tree structures, 1993 (Bethesda, MD: National Library of Medicine, 1993) p. 835.

Figure 4-4. Permuted *MeSH*

Each significant term in a subject heading *or* cross-reference is listed alphabetically, e.g., QUALITY OF HEALTH CARE would be listed under **Quality**, **Health**, and **Care** followed by appropriate MeSH term(s).

CARE

ACCEPTABILITY OF HEALTH CARE see PATIENT ACCEPTANCE OF HEALTH CARE
ACCESS TO HEALTH CARE see HEALTH SERVICES ACCESSIBILITY
AFTER CARE
AGENCY FOR HEALTH CARE POLICY AND RESEARCH see UNITED STATES AGENCY FOR HEALTH CARE POLICY AND RESEARCH
AMBULATORY CARE
AMBULATORY CARE FACILITIES
AMBULATORY CARE FACILITIES, HOSPITAL see OUTPATIENT CLINICS, HOSPITAL
AMBULATORY CARE INFORMATION SYSTEMS
ANIMAL CARE COMMITTEES see ANIMAL WELFARE
ASSESSMENT OF HEALTH CARE NEEDS see HEALTH SERVICES NEEDS AND DEMAND
BEREAVEMENT CARE see HOSPICE CARE
BUSINESS COALITIONS (HEALTH CARE) see HEALTH CARE COALITIONS
CANCER CARE FACILITIES
CANCER CARE UNITS see ONCOLOGY SERVICE, HOSPITAL
CARDIAC CARE FACILITIES
CHILD CARE

PREOPERATIVE CARE
PREPAID DENTAL CARE see INSURANCE, DENTAL
PRIMARY CARE PHYSICIANS see PHYSICIANS, FAMILY
PRIMARY HEALTH CARE
PRIMARY NURSING CARE
PROCESS ASSESSMENT (HEALTH CARE)
PROGRESSIVE PATIENT CARE
QUALITY ASSESSMENT, HEALTH CARE see QUALITY ASSURANCE, HEALTH CARE
QUALITY ASSURANCE, HEALTH CARE
QUALITY OF HEALTH CARE
RATIONING, HEALTH CARE see HEALTH CARE RATIONI 'G
RESPIRATORY CARE UNITS
RESPITE CARE
SELF CARE
ROOMING–IN CARE
SELF–CARE (REHABILITATION) see ACTIVITIES OF DAILY LIVING
SELF–CARE UNITS
TERMINAL CARE
UNITED STATES AGENCY FOR HEALTH CARE POLICY AND RESEARCH
UNITED STATES HEALTH CARE FINANCING ADMINISTRATION

QUALITY

AIR QUALITY, INDOOR see AIR POLLUTION, INDOOR
INDOOR AIR QUALITY see AIR POLLUTION, INDOOR
MANAGEMENT QUALITY CIRCLES
QUALITY, ACCESS, EVALUATION (NON MESH)
QUALITY ASSESSMENT, HEALTH CARE see QUALITY ASSURANCE, HEALTH CARE
QUALITY ASSURANCE, HEALTH CARE
QUALITY CIRCLES see MANAGEMENT QUALITY CIRCLES
QUALITY CONTROL
QUALITY OF HEALTH CARE
QUALITY OF LIFE
UTILIZATION AND QUALITY CONTROL PEER REVIEW ORGANIZATIONS see PROFESSIONAL REVIEW ORGANIZATIONS
VOICE QUALITY

HEALTH

ABUSE OF HEALTH SERVICES see HEALTH SERVICES MISUSE
ACCEPTABILITY OF HEALTH CARE see PATIENT ACCEPTANCE OF HEALTH CARE
ACCESS TO HEALTH CARE see HEALTH SERVICES ACCESSIBILITY
ACCESSIBILITY OF HEALTH SERVICES see HEALTH SERVICES ACCESSIBILITY
ACQUISITION, HEALTH FACILITY see HEALTH FACILITY MERGER
ADOLESCENT HEALTH SERVICES
AGENCY FOR HEALTH CARE POLICY AND RESEARCH see UNITED STATES AGENCY FOR HEALTH CARE POLICY AND RESEARCH
ALCOHOL, DRUG ABUSE, AND MENTAL HEALTH ADMINISTRATION (U.S.) see UNITED STATES ALCOHOL, DRUG ABUSE, AND MENTAL HEALTH ADMINISTRATION
ALLIED HEALTH OCCUPATIONS
ALLIED HEALTH PERSONNEL
AREA HEALTH EDUCATION CENTERS
ASSESSMENT OF HEALTH CARE NEEDS see HEALTH SERVICES NEEDS AND DEMAND
ATTITUDE OF HEALTH PERSONNEL
ATTITUDE TO HEALTH
AUTOMATED MULTIPHASIC HEALTH TESTING see MULTIPHASIC SCREENING
AVAILABILITY OF HEALTH SERVICES see HEALTH SERVICES ACCESSIBILITY
BUSINESS COALITIONS (HEALTH CARE) see HEALTH CARE COALITIONS
CATASTROPHIC HEALTH INSURANCE see INSURANCE, MAJOR MEDICAL
CATCHMENT AREA (HEALTH)
CENTERS FOR HEALTH PLANNING see HEALTH PLANNING ORGANIZATIONS

PUBLIC HEALTH ADMINISTRATION
PUBLIC HEALTH DENTISTRY
PUBLIC HEALTH NURSING
PUBLIC HEALTH PRACTICE (NON MESH)
PUBLIC HEALTH SCHOOLS see SCHOOLS, PUBLIC HEALTH
PUBLIC HEALTH SERVICE (U.S.) see UNITED STATES PUBLIC HEALTH SERVICE
PUBLIC HEALTH SURVEILLANCE see POPULATION SURVEILLANCE
QUALITY ASSESSMENT, HEALTH CARE see QUALITY ASSURANCE, HEALTH CARE
QUALITY ASSURANCE, HEALTH CARE
QUALITY OF HEALTH CARE
RADIOLOGIC HEALTH (NON MESH)
RATIONING, HEALTH CARE see HEALTH CARE RATIONING
REGIONAL HEALTH PLANNING
REIMBURSEMENT, HEALTH INSURANCE see INSURANCE, HEALTH, REIMBURSEMENT
RESEARCH, HEALTH SERVICES see HEALTH SERVICES RESEARCH
RURAL HEALTH
SCHOOL HEALTH SERVICES
SCHOOLS, HEALTH OCCUPATIONS
SCHOOLS, PUBLIC HEALTH
STATE HEALTH PLANNING AND DEVELOPMENT AGENCIES
STATE HEALTH PLANNING, UNITED STATES see HEALTH PLANNING
STATE HEALTH PLANS
STATEWIDE HEALTH COORDINATING COUNCILS see HEALTH PLANNING COUNCILS
STUDENT HEALTH SERVICES
STUDENTS, HEALTH OCCUPATIONS
SUBSIDIES, HEALTH PLANNING see HEALTH PLANNING SUPPORT
TECHNICAL ASSISTANCE FOR HEALTH PLANNING see HEALTH PLANNING TECHNICAL ASSISTANCE
UNITED STATES AGENCY FOR HEALTH CARE POLICY AND RESEARCH

National Library of Medicine. Permuted medical subject headings, 1993 (Bethesda, MD: National Library of Medicine, 1993) pp. 80-1, 226-8, 420.

views of reported known or published cases; and state of the art reviews" [5]. A separate author index was available until 1980. The *BMR* first appeared as a separate publication. Its cumulation (volume 6, 1961) represents review articles from the 1955-1959 *Current List of Medical Literature* and from the *Cumulated Index Medicus (CIM)*, volume 1, 1960; however, editing procedures for the cumulation resulted in some references being eliminated. Subsequent volumes 7-12, 1962-67 contain references to review articles from the previous years' *CIM*, volumes 2-7, 1961-66. The *BMR*, now a regular feature of both the monthly and cumulated *Index Medicus*, has listed the current year's review articles since the *CIM*, volume 8, 1967, and the monthly *IM*, volume 9, no. 1, Jan. 1968. These were also separately published in five-year cumulations covering 1966-1970, 1971-1975, and 1976-1980.

The MEDLARS files are also used to produce the *Abridged Index Medicus (AIM)*, volume 1- , 1970- . Designed to be used by the practicing physician, *AIM* provides citations to 117 English-language clinical journals. The format is similar to that of *Index Medicus*, with both author and subject indexes. MeSH terms are used, with the modification that articles are only listed under main headings in the monthly issues and under main heading/subheadings when appropriate in the annual *Cumulated Abridged Index Medicus*. *AIM* is an especially useful index for the smaller health sciences library where the focus is on the need for clinical literature rather than the exhaustive research journal coverage of *Index Medicus*. Although *AIM* is still published, librarians and health professionals are encouraged to access this literature online, either directly or through assist programs such as GRATEFUL MED, BRS/ Colleague, PaperChase, or DIALOG Medical Connection (*see* Chapter 5).

OTHER MEDICAL INDEXES AND ABSTRACTS

4.2 *Excerpta Medica*. Amsterdam, The Netherlands, Excerpta Medica, 1947- . 46 sections.

4.3 *Medical Socioeconomic Research Sources*. Chicago, Archive Library Department of the American Medical Association, Vols. 1-9, 1971-1979. Formerly: *Index to Medical Socioeconomic Literature*. Vols. 1-9, 1962-1970.

Excerpta Medica (EM) is a major abstracting service for medical journals. Its scope is primarily human medicine and the basic sciences related to this field. While allied medical subjects (dentistry, nursing, psychology, veterinary medicine, etc.) appear in the sections, they are not the primary subject fields abstracted. *EM* covers more than 4,500 journals, 3,500 of which are regularly scanned. These represent 95% of the *Excerpta Medica* references, with monographs and dissertations making up the remaining 5%. The abstracts appear in one or more of the more than forty subject sections of *EM*. Each section has its own editor who selects the articles that will appear in that section and, further, decides whether the references will be abstracted for the printed *EM* publication or just be indexed and appear in the EM database under the section's classification (EMCLAS) number. Sixty percent of the references appear in at least one printed *Excerpta Medica* section. The remaining 40% of the file is available only through online searching of EMBASE, the *Excerpta Medica* database. The sections arrange the references, with abstracts, in a classified (subject) order within each section, with author and detailed subject indexes. Two of the *Excerpta Medica* sections, *Drug Literature Index* and *Adverse Reactions Titles*, are indexes only and do not provide abstracts.

From 1974-1990, subjects were indexed using *EM*'s controlled vocabulary, *MAster LIst of MEdical indexing Terms* (MALIMET). The MALIMET vocabulary began as a loosely controlled vocabulary of more than 250,000 terms. In 1991, the *EMTREE Thesaurus*, an integrated vocabulary of 35,000 medical and drug terms, was published, merging MALIMET, medical EMCLAS, drug EMCLAS, and EMTAG indexing systems into a single thesaurus [6].

Even with the new *EMTREE Thesaurus*, Excerpta Medica's *Guide to the Classification and Indexing System* (Princeton, NJ: Excerpta Medica, 1988) is essential reading for anyone beginning a manual search of *Excerpta Medica*. The introductory section provides general information about the *Guide* and examples of how to use it in preparing a search strategy. The second section provides a breakdown of the Excerpta Medica Classification (EMCLAS) system with contents of each of the printed *EM* sections, 1-52, followed by brief listings for the literature indexes that appeared from 1975-1977. The third section is an index to EMCLAS and is primarily a guide for online searchers in identifying appropriate classification numbers for searching EMBASE. Section four is the Excerpta Medica Item Index System (EMTAGS) and includes all codes used since 1969. Scope notes are included for more effective manual and online searching. The "Guide to Subject Index Terminology" section in the 1983 edition has been replaced by *Mini-MALIMET* (1st ed., 1986), which lists the 20,000 most frequently used MALIMET terms. The *Guide*, in conjunction with *Mini-MALIMET*, should prove useful for both online and manual searching for the time periods covered.

Because of its detailed indexing vocabulary, *Excerpta Medica* is often useful in locating articles on very narrow topics that do not have a specific enough subject approach in *Index Medicus*. Its abstracts are also helpful for providing English summaries of non-English-language articles. These are useful in helping a researcher decide whether the article should be obtained or translated.

On the negative side, *Excerpta Medica* is an extremely costly service for a library to purchase, house, and maintain. However, subject sections can be purchased separately, allowing smaller specialized libraries to purchase only those sections useful to their primary clientele.

Medical Socioeconomic Research Sources (Med Soc), a quarterly publication that cumulated annually, was produced by the Division of Library and Archival Services staff of the AMA in cooperation with its Center for Health Services Research and Development and Electronic Data Processing Section. The index selectively covered English-language books, journal articles, pamphlets, unpublished speeches, theses, and selected newspaper articles in the sociology and economics of medicine. Other specific areas covered include education, ethics, international relations, legislation, political science, public health, religion, and statistics related to medicine.

The main index lists citations under subject headings based on *MeSH* but adapted to the subject areas covered in *Med Soc*. Broad subjects are arranged in a hierarchical arrangement using subheadings. The author index lists the citation under the first author's name, with cross-references from the second and third authors only. The index is helpful in identifying articles with statistical information for the time period covered. It is also useful for locating material from less technical sources for less sophisticated medical library users. Unfortunately, this index ceased publication in 1979. It was available online along with several AMA-produced reference titles, e.g., *Current Medical Information and Terminology (CMIT)*, through AMA/NET from 1981 until 1991, when the AMA dropped AMA/NET. Access to medical socioeconomic information is now limited to those sources covered by *Index Medicus, Excerpta Medica,* and *Hospital Literature Index* and their electronic counterparts.

Nursing Indexes

4.4 *International Nursing Index.* New York, American Journal of Nursing Company, in cooperation with the National Library of Medicine, Vol. 1- , 1966- . Quarterly.

4.5 *Cumulative Index to Nursing and Allied Health Literature.* Glendale, CA, Glendale Adventist Medical Center, Vol. 22- , 1977- . Bimonthly. Formerly: *Cumulative Index to Nursing Literature*, vols. 1-21, 1956-1976.

4.6 Henderson, V. *Nursing Studies Index; an annotated guide to reported studies, research in progress, research methods, and historical materials in periodicals, books and pamphlets in English.* Vols. 1-4, 1900-1959. Philadelphia, PA, Lippincott, 1963-1972.

The *International Nursing Index (INI)* appears quarterly and has a format identical to that of *Index Medicus*, with subject and author indexes. A *Nursing Thesaurus* (supplementary to *MeSH*) is used for the subject index. This annotated list of subject headings, as well as a list of the more than 270 journals indexed (not all of which are indexed by *Index Medicus*), appear in the annual cumulation.

Journal coverage is international in scope and, in addition to the citations from nursing journals, includes references to nursing articles from nonnursing journals gleaned from the MEDLARS system. Original signed articles, editorials of national and international interest, and biographies and obituaries of substance comprise the coverage, as well as reports of national and international organizations and nursing dissertations. Special sections in the index include a "List of Nursing Books" and a "List of Publications of Organizations and Agencies." From 1986 through 1990, *INI* included in the annual cumulation a "Nursing Citation Index" section, provided by the Institute for Scientific Information, following the format of the *Science Citation Index*.

The *Cumulative Index to Nursing and Allied Health Literature (CINAHL)* appears in five bimonthly issues (called *Nursing and Allied Health Index*) and a cumulated annual volume. It covers the English-language nursing and allied health literature. It has separate author and subject indexes. (Prior to 1967, authors and subjects were in a single alphabetical listing.)

In preparation for providing online access to its index, *CINAHL* published a *Transition Guide* (Glendale, CA: Glendale Adventist Medical Center, 1983) to *CINAHL* subject headings. This subject headings list has been expanded and refined annually. Resembling *MeSH*, the list provides an alphabetic list, a tree structure, and permuted listing of terms. The subject listing appears in the annual cumulation and includes scope notes, date a term entered the vocabulary, and cross-references.

The index format remains the same. Many references to journal articles indicate the type of article in parentheses following the citation, e.g., "research," "review," or "case study." Nursing students often find these notations quite helpful. Separate indexes provide references to new books from more than thirty health sciences publishers and nursing dissertations submitted to University Microfilms International (UMI) for *Dissertation Abstracts International*.

More than 330 nursing and allied health journals and more than a dozen journals in health sciences librarianship are regularly scanned, using essentially the same criteria as *INI*. In addition, *CINAHL* indexes all serials published by the American Nurses Association, the National League for Nursing, and the Division of Nursing of the Department of Health and Human Services (DHHS). Additional journals covered in an issue are listed when they have been indexed, for example, popular and news magazines such as *Newsweek, Parents'*, and *McCalls*.

CINAHL regularly includes approximately 120 journals not indexed in *INI*. On the other hand, it does not have the nonnursing and foreign journal coverage that *INI* gets from MEDLARS. Discussion in the literature [7] highlights two ways of looking at the journal coverage overlap, while Prime [8] points out the unique coverage of each index. The two indexes complement each other, even though the core nursing literature is generally covered by both. *CINAHL*, however, appears bimonthly rather than quarterly and tends to get articles indexed more rapidly.

The *Nursing Studies Index*, compiled by the Yale University School of Nursing Index staff, provides retrospective coverage of the English-language nursing literature from 1900 to 1959 in a subject arrangement. Subjects are subdivided by both geographic subheadings and general subheadings such as evaluations, manuals, etc. An author index is also provided.

Dental Indexes and Abstracts

4.7 *Index to Dental Literature*. Chicago, American Dental Association and National Library of Medicine, 1962- . Quarterly.

4.8 *Dental Abstracts; a selection of world dental literature*. Chicago, American Dental Association, Vol. 1- , 1956- . Bimonthly. (1956-1989, Monthly).

4.9 *Oral Research Abstracts*. Chicago, American Dental Association, Vols. 1-13, 1966-1978.

The *Index to Dental Literature (IDL)* is the primary index to dental literature. It is international in scope and includes both dental journals and references to related articles from nondental journals in the MEDLARS files. Each quarterly issue is cumulative and lists all journals indexed therein. The fourth issue is an annual bound volume.

IDL has been published in cooperation with the National Library of Medicine since 1965. It was previously published as *Index of the Periodical Dental Literature*, beginning with the 1839-1875 volume. Subsequent volumes came out in various cumulations and only covered the English language until 1961. Arrangement varied through the years with the pattern being 1836-1938, subject listing with an author index; 1939-1964, author-subject listing; 1965 to date, subject arrangement with an author index. The latter follows the format of *Index Medicus*.

Criteria for inclusion of an article are similar to those for the nursing indexes: original signed articles, editorials of national and international interest, reports of national and international organizations, and selected bibliographies. A list of dental descriptors gives cross-references and refers the user to *MeSH* for a complete subject heading listing. MeSH subheadings with definitions are included but are called "qualifiers." The subject index and the author index are in the same format as *Index Medicus*. Separate listings of dental books published and dental dissertations and theses arranged by author, country and institution, and subject are also included, as well as a "Bibliography of Dental Reviews." The preface gives a concise explanation of the index, how it is constructed, and how to use it.

Dental Abstracts appeared monthly through 1989. It is now a bimonthly publication that abstracts approximately 1,000 journal articles a year from the world's literature. It provides a classified listing by broad subject and gives author and subject indexes with the last issue of the year. There is a four- to seven-month time lag between the publication of an article in a journal and its appearance in *Dental Abstracts*. Another distinct disadvantage of this publication is that it does not provide a list of the journals it abstracts.

Oral Research Abstracts appeared monthly but was broader in scope than *Dental Abstracts* and included both dental and nondental journals. Its purpose was "to bring the facts to their [dentists'] desks and permit selective reading of original reports" [9]. Approximately 7,200 signed abstracts appeared annually, taken from more than 1,000 journals (not listed with *Dental Abstracts*) and patents from world literature. There is a classified arrangement with an author index in the monthly issues and subject and author indexes in the annual cumulated volumes. Abstracts are more descriptive than critical.

Hospital Indexes and Abstracts

4.10 *Hospital Literature Index*. Chicago, American Hospital Association, in cooperation with the National Library of Medicine, Vol. 11- , 1955-. Quarterly. Formerly: *Hospital Periodical Literature Index*, vols. 1-10, 1945-1954.

4.11 *Hospital Abstracts; a monthly survey of world literature*. London, Department of Health and Social Security, Jan. 1961-Dec. 1984. Monthly. Prepared by: *Ministry of Health*, Jan. 1961-Dec. 1962.

4.12 *Abstracts of Health Care Management Studies*. Ann Arbor, MI, University of Michigan, Cooperative Information Center for Health Care Management Studies, Vols. 15-23, 1979-July 1987. Annual. Formerly: *Abstracts of Hospital Management Studies*, vols. 1-14, 1964-78.

The *Hospital Literature Index* (*HLI*) has gone through several changes prior to its present format as a quarterly publication, which has been produced in cooperation with NLM since 1978 using the MEDLARS Health Planning and Administration database. Earlier titles—*Index of Current Hos-*

pital Literature, volumes 1-10, 1945-1954; *Hospital Periodical Literature Index,* volumes 11-13(1), 1955-June 1957; and *Hospital Literature Index,* 1957-1958— were regularly compiled into six five-year cumulations as *Cumulative Index to Hospital Literature* (1945-49, 1950-54, 1955-59, 1960-64, 1965-69, 1970-74) and a final multiyear volume for 1975-77. Subsequent cumulations under MEDLARS appear annually, similar to those of the *International Nursing Index.*

The *Hospital Literature Index* covers English-language journal literature related to the administrative aspects of the delivery of health care in hospitals, health centers, health maintenance organizations (HMOs) and other group practice facilities. Also included are articles related to nursing homes, rehabilitation centers, etc. Clinical medicine and the clinical aspects of patient care are not covered in this index, but articles on the quality of patient care can be found. The present format of *HLI* is like that of *Index Medicus,* with citations listed directly under the subject headings as well as by the first author's name in the author index. MeSH terms (with an expanded vocabulary in hospital management and planning) are now used for subject headings in *HLI.* This superseded Alice Dunlap's *Hospital Literature Subject Headings* (Chicago: American Hospital Association, 2d ed., 1977), which should be used for subject access to the cumulative indexes, 1945-1977. The publication, *Hospital Literature Subject Headings Transition Guide to Medical Subject Headings* (Chicago: American Hospital Association, 1978), was designed to aid in the shift in subject heading coverage made necessary by conversion to the MEDLARS system. Now the *MeSH* thesaurus should be used.

In addition to the primary subject and author indexes, *HLI* provides a list of journals indexed by journal title abbreviation. A special section provides listings of books, monographs, and journals recently received by the AHA Resource Center, which includes the Asa S. Bacon Memorial Library of the American Hospital Association, the Center for Hospital and Healthcare Administration History, and the Hospital Literature Service.

Hospital Abstracts, a monthly British publication, provided abstracts of articles on all aspects of hospitals and hospital administration through 1984. Indexing was selective for nonmedical journals. Although only 1,825 abstracts were provided in 1982, more than half of the journals were not covered in *Index Medicus.* References are arranged in broad subject categories and by hospital departments. The cumulated annual volumes have both subject and author indexes.

Abstracts of Health Care Management Studies provides an approach to a somewhat different body of literature. Published annually (from 1964 until 1987) by the Cooperative Information Center for Health Care Management Studies of the University of Michigan, it provides abstracts of management, planning, and public policies related to the delivery of health care. Both published and unpublished studies, as well as those with limited distribution were abstracted.

The abstracts are arranged in a classified format of forty categories with author and subject indexes. Signed abstracts include bibliographic information and availability and ordering information for unpublished studies. A specialized index, the SOurce of Reference INdex (SORIN), appeared in the 1979 volume but has been subsequently dropped. SORIN lists the sources of abstracted studies, including research agencies, sites of studies, universities, foundations, sponsoring government agencies, and journals. A list of journals gives routinely scanned sources with publishers, addresses, etc. A microfilm index, which was dropped beginning with the 1983 volume, listed those items available in that format from University Microfilms International. Publisher and corporate author indexes were added in 1983.

These latter two sources complemented the coverage of *Hospital Literature Index* and it is unfortunate that they ceased publication and were never made available online.

OTHER RELATED INDEXES AND ABSTRACTS

4.13 *Biological Abstracts.* Philadelphia, PA, BioSciences Information Services, Vol. 1- , 1926- . Biweekly.

4.14 *Biological Abstracts/RRM (Reports, Reviews and Meetings).* Philadelphia, PA, BioSciences Information Service. Vol. 22- , 1982- . Bimonthly. (Monthly, vols. 18-21, 1980-81.) Formerly: *Bioresearch Titles,* vols. 1-2, 1965-66; *BioResearch Index,* vols. 3-17, 1967-79.

Biological Abstracts (BA) and *Biological Abstracts/RRM (BA/RRM)* should be used in conjunction for searching all types of literature in the life sciences. BioSciences Information Service (BIOSIS) has designed them so that the same reference is rarely listed in both. Each biweekly issue of *BA* contains abstracts of original article research papers (arranged under approximately 580 broad subject specialties). The two semiannual cumulations abstract more than 149,000 articles from 8,000 periodicals each year [10]. Now appearing semimonthly, *BA/RRM* indexes additional research reports not in *BA,* as well as symposia, reviews, bibliographies, book chapters, and selected government reports, providing a content summary for each. New book synopses will appear at the beginning of each issue as well. More than 113,000 citations appear annually. A complete list of coverage, plus a description of how to search the indexes, is provided at the end of each cumulated index.

Both publications have the same kinds of index access, with reference numbers referring to the section with the bibliographic citation. These include

The Author Index, which lists up to the first ten authors.
The Biological Abstracts Subject Index in Context (BASIC), a computer-permuted KWIC index that uses the author's title augmented by significant words from the abstract and article. Foreign-language titles are translated into English. This type of index, without a controlled vocabulary, requires the user to prepare a list of as many synonyms as possible to search a subject thoroughly.
The Biosystematic Index, which allows a search to be made on a taxonomic category.
The Concept Index (formerly Cross Index), which is an index by the subject concepts used in arranging the abstracts. Although an abstract and its reference are listed under only one subject concept, it will be listed by reference number under all relevant concepts in this index.
The Generic Index, which provides access by Latin name to all organisms, except viruses, gleaned from authors' titles or keywords extracted from texts.

A thorough search of these five indexes in either *BA* or *BA/RRM* is complex; however, BIOSIS provides helpful guides to their use in the introduction to *BA* and the *Guide to the Use of Biological Abstracts*. Even so, *BA* is, in most cases, easier to search online than manually.

4.15 *Chemical Abstracts.* Columbus, OH, Chemical Abstracts Service, Vol. 1- , 1907- . Weekly.

Chemical Abstracts (CA) provides international coverage of the chemical literature from more than 14,000 scientific and technical journals, as well as conference proceedings, congresses and symposia, technical reports, dissertations, new books, announcements, and patents from twenty-six countries. Approximately one-third of the literature is biochemical. Abstracts are arranged in eighty sections; sections 1-34 include biochemistry and organic chemistry, while sections 35-80 cover macromolecular chemistry, applied chemistry and chemical engineering, and physical and analytical chemistry. These broad section categories are issued in alternate weeks and cumulate into two volumes (twenty-six issues per volume) each year.
The indexes to *CA* are numerous and complex. Weekly indexes include

An author index to authors, patentees, and patent assignees.

An alphabetic keyword index to works and phrases from titles, abstracts, and texts.

A patent index arranged numerically by country.

A patent concordance that cross-references a patent either applied for or granted in different countries, with the first reference in *CA* to the patent dealing with the invention.

Only the first reference to a given patent is abstracted. Volume indexes (semiannual) include the cumulated weekly numerical patent and patent concordances. Other volume indexes are newly constructed. These include an author index, general subject index, chemical substance index, formula index, and index to ring systems. Use of the general subject and substance volume indexes must be preceded by a study of the *Index Guide*, which lists entry points to the volume indexes published at the beginning of each collective period (five years) as well as indexing policies for the time period. The most recent *Index Guide* (March 1992) is available for the most recent collective period, 1987-91. Supplements to the *Index Guide* are published annually and are cumulative between collective periods. Use of the *Index Guide* is essential to proper subject and chemical subject searching of *CA*, due to the policy of controlled compound naming used by the Chemical Abstracts Service (CAS). In addition, a computer-based CAS Chemical Registry System assigns a unique "registry number" to a chemical substance, identifying it by description of its structure, including its stereochemical characteristics. The *CA Registry Handbook* and its supplements provide access by registry numbers to *CA* index names and molecular formulas, thus providing entry points to the substance and formula indexes.

4.16 *Science Citation Index.* Philadelphia, PA, Institute for Scientific Information, 1961- . Bimonthly.

The *Science Citation Index (SCI)* is an interdisciplinary index, with 54% of its coverage being literature in the life sciences and clinical practice. Its uniqueness lies in the indexing approach it presents. In addition to an alphabetical author index, which includes a corporate index called the Source Index and a permuted keyword subject index called the Permuted Subject Index, it provides a Citation Index listing the bibliographic references that are cited in current articles listed in the Source Index. The Citation Index also includes an anonymous citation index and a patent citation index. References are indexed from approximately 3,200 source publications, approximately 125 of which are monographic series. The index appears bimonthly (originally it was a quarterly publication) with annual and five-year cumulations. The latter makes manual retrospective searching relatively convenient.

The indexing of citations and their subsequent searching have definite advantages, but this approach also has some pitfalls. It is useful for locating current information on an obscure new topic not easily defined by the controlled vocabulary of *Index Medicus* or even *Excerpta Medica*. It is also quite useful in updating references to an author's research or to the current uses of a specific technique, or in identifying how well received or accepted an author has become. It can identify references to a topic in literature outside the primary discipline of the original author. On the other hand, cited references have their disadvantages. At present, citations are not checked for accuracy, and a miscited article may go undetected. The author's name may be cited inconsistently, using only one initial (either first or second) instead of two. For thoroughness, all possible permutations of an author's name should be checked in the index. In addition, the year, volume, or page numbers of an article may be miscited. Transposition of any of these numbers can easily occur.

It should be noted that only first authors are cited. Additional authors' names are listed in the Source Index with cross-reference to the first author's name where the full citation is listed.

The *Science Citation Index Guide and Lists of Source Publications*, published annually, provides hints on citation searching and sample citations, citation indexing, a list of publications indexed, as well as essays on the Institute for Scientific Information.

4.17 *Psychological Abstracts*. Lancaster, PA, American Psychological Association, Vol. 1- , 1927- . Monthly.

Psychological Abstracts (PA) appeared monthly with two numbered bibliographic volumes and volume indexes a year through 1983. Since 1984, *PA* appears monthly in a single bibliographic volume with an annual cumulated index. More than 1,100 journals, technical reports, and monographs are abstracted from the world literature of psychology and its related disciplines. Some journals are selectively abstracted and may not appear in a given volume of *PA*. Dissertations from *Dissertation Abstracts International* are indexed but not abstracted.

The nonevaluative abstracts (some are signed) are arranged under sixteen major classified categories. Author and brief subject indexes are provided in each monthly issue, with an expanded and integrated subject index cumulated every six months.

Subject headings used in the subject indexes are assigned from the 4,000-word *Thesaurus of Psychological Index Terms* (Washington, DC: American Psychological Association, 1991, 6th ed.). Only subject headings and their cross-references used for citations in an issue are listed in the monthly subject indexes. Three-year cumulated indexes are available through 1983, and reference numbers to abstracts are consecutive within each volume. It is, therefore, important to note the volume and year when using these cumulative indexes. Starting in 1984, *PA* began issuing annual author and subject cumulations.

A significant amount of clinically related material is abstracted in *PA*. It is especially useful for locating reference to the psychological aspects of diseases and subsequent behavioral changes.

CURRENT AWARENESS SERVICES

Even with the aid of computers to compile and format the printed indexing and abstracting journals, there is a significant time lag between publication of a journal article and its appearance in an index or abstract. As a result, several rapid current awareness periodicals have been developed. The Institute for Scientific Information's (ISI) weekly *Current Contents* journals are the most notable. In the health sciences, four are particularly popular:

4.18 *Current Contents: Agriculture, Biology, and Environmental Sciences.* Philadelphia, PA, Institute for Scientific Information, Vol. 1- , 1970- . Weekly.

4.19 *Current Contents: Social and Behavioral Sciences.* Philadelphia, PA, Institute for Scientific Information, Vol. 1- , 1969- . Weekly.

4.20 *Current Contents: Clinical Practice.* Philadelphia, PA, Institute for Scientific Information, Vol. 1- , 1973- . Weekly.

4.21 *Current Contents: Life Sciences.* Philadelphia, PA, Institute for Scientific Information, Vol. 1- , 1958- . Weekly.

Current Contents provides copies of the table of contents pages of current journals within weeks of their publication. (Not infrequently, *Current Contents* arrives in a library before the journal itself, most frequently for foreign publications.) Author and keyword subject indexes refer to the *Current Contents* pages on which the reference appears. Also indicated is the beginning page number of the article in the table of contents for that journal, thus providing rapid access to the reference.

Excerpta Medica Foundation has also entered the current awareness field with *Core Journals* in the fields of cardiology, clinical neurology, dermatology, gastroenterology, obstetrics and gynecology, ophthalmology, and pediatrics. Combining the table of contents feature of *Current Contents* with abstracts from specialized subject journals, the *Core Journals* provide abstracts within six weeks of publication for articles within these specialties. The *Core Journals* are published monthly (11 issues a year) and provide no indexes. They appear to be designed for individual clinicians and researchers, rather than for libraries.

There are many specialized indexes a library should consider carrying to satisfy the needs of its primary user population. This chapter has highlighted only the major ones in the health sciences. Consideration of new and additional indexes and abstracting journals should be weighed against a library's present holdings to determine if the new work(s) will be of significant value to add to the collection. Some of these considerations are timeliness of publication, provision of access to materials not indexed elsewhere, and provision of unique access approaches (e.g., report numbers).

REFERENCES

1. See also: Broadman E. The development of medical bibliography. Chicago: Medical Library Association, 1954;115-23.

2. Kunz J. Index Medicus, century of medical citation. JAMA 1979 Jan 26;241:387-90.

3. Austin CF. MEDLARS 1963-1967. Bethesda, MD: National Library of Medicine, 1968.

4. National Library of Medicine. The principles of MEDLARS. Bethesda, MD: National Institutes of Health, 1970.

5. Introduction. Index Medicus 1993 Jan;33(no. 1, pt.2):xi.

6. EMTREE thesaurus. Amsterdam and New York: Excerpta Medica, 1991.

7. Foreman GE. Journal coverage in the nursing indexes: International Nursing Index and Cumulative Index to Nursing and Allied Health Literature. Med Ref Serv Q 1983 Spring;2:1-5.

8. Prime EE. Letter to the Editor. Med Ref Serv Q 1983 Spring; 2:91-4.

9. Oral Res Absts 1966:2.

10. A study in BIOSIS preview memo (v. 1, no. 2, July 1979) notes that 78.8% of Index Medicus journals are included in BA. This, of course, refers to journal coverage but not necessarily articles indexed.

READINGS

BioSciences Information Service. Guide to the indexes for biological abstracts and bioresearch index. Philadelphia: BioSciences Information Service of Biological Abstracts, 1972.

CAS printed access tools, a workbook. Washington, DC: American Chemical Society, 1981.

King MM, King LS. Guide to searching the biological literature. Boca Raton, FL: Science Media, a div. of J. Jusey Association, 1978. (slides and audiotape)

Poyner RK. Time lag in four indexing services. Spec Lib 1982 April;13:142-50.

Science citation index guide and lists of source publications. Philadelphia: Institute for Scientific Information. (annual)

CHAPTER 5

Electronic Bibliographic Databases

Jo Anne Boorkman

> We are moving rather rapidly and quite inevitably toward a paper-less society. Advances in computer science and in communications technology allow us to conceive of a global system in which reports of research and development activities are composed, published, disseminated, and used in a completely electronic mode [1].

The above statement, written in 1978, has yet to be fulfilled. However, libraries are moving closer to that vision in the 1990s. For health sciences libraries, the advent of the use of computers in retrieving references to the medical literature online began in 1968 with the SUNY/BIOMEDICAL Communications Network, forerunner of Bibliographic Retrieval Service (BRS). That was followed by the implementation of the National Library of Medicine's AIM-TWX (*Abridged Index Medicus* via TeletypeWriter eXchange) project in the spring of 1971. Developing from this project, MEDLINE (*MEDical Literature Analysis and Retrieval System*, or *MEDLARS onLINE*), containing citations from the *Index Medicus, Index to Dental Literature,* and *International Nursing Index,* became available online in the fall of 1971 [2]. Today there are hundreds of bibliographic databases that have their counterparts in printed indexes and abstracts. A growing number of bibliographic and nonbibliographic reference tools are produced only in electronic form.

Other reference tools, such as *American Men and Women of Science;* indexes of medical textbooks, e.g., Comprehensive Core Medical Library (CCML) from BRS; and entire texts of journals, e.g., those published by the American Chemical Society, have an established record as full-text online files. More recently some are appearing as portable files in disk and CD-ROM formats. While there is rapid growth and variety in the types of information available online and in portable formats, this chapter will concentrate on the bibliographic databases, which are still the primary databases accessed by searchers, and increasingly by end users, in health sciences libraries.

The computer technology that makes it possible for indexing and abstracting services to facilitate access to the rapidly growing periodical literature also makes it possible to manipulate the bibliographic information in a variety of ways. As a result, the data files can be used to extract references for individualized demand bibliographies on a variety of topics.

Four major vendors—BRS, CompuServ, DIALOG, and the National Library of Medicine (NLM)—provide access to the majority of online bibliographic databases used by health sciences libraries in the United States [3]. SDC Search Service ORBIT, cited by Werner [4] in 1979, no longer offers the primary health sciences databases used by most health sciences libraries. Each vendor provides detailed user manuals on how to search its systems as well as specific information about searching the various databases. In addition, some of the database producers have provided manuals describing their indexing policies and special features of the unit record (all the bibliographic and descriptive components used to describe an entry in a database: author[s], title, journal, keywords, page numbers, etc.). These manuals are essential reading for anyone actually searching the databases; because this material is detailed and varies from database to database, there will be no attempt to cover it here.

According to the 1979 survey by Werner [5], the majority of health sciences libraries provide online bibliographic searches through the reference department. This pattern has not changed [6] and, in fact, has intensified with the introduction of locally mounted databases and microcomputer-based CD-ROMs. In smaller institutions the entire staff provides the service. This chapter will, therefore, discuss the databases most widely used as reference tools in the health sciences. Features of each will be discussed as they relate to their function in reference and as they complement the printed reference collection.

For mediated searches, whether or not the user should be present while the search is being processed by the librarian has been a matter of considerable discussion [7-8]. A survey of actual practice reveals that the majority of searches in the health sciences are processed by librarians without the end user present, and only rarely is the user allowed to run the search with or without assistance [9]. However, this trend is changing as a growing number of individuals have personal computers and are interested in learning to do their own searching. A more recent survey, albeit in the social sciences setting, indicated a 77% preference for having the client present so "that the search can be refined...during the search" [10]. The author's survey revealed intense interest on the part of library clients in doing their own searches over locally available databases, whether mounted on minicomputers, mainframes, or on PC-based CD-ROMs. Nevertheless, it is essential that the librarian/searcher conduct a thorough reference interview to ascertain the full needs of the user [11-12]. In addition to a thorough reference interview, the librarian plays a key role in instruction in the use of the appropriate database(s) when the client wants to perform his or her own search.

Often an individual will come to the library for a computer search when the information needed can be found readily by using more traditional reference tools. The user may also request a specific database, such as MEDLINE, when other databases may be better suited to the request or should be considered in addition to MEDLINE. Proper interviewing can suggest the appropriate solution to the user's need and save the librarian and user both time and money, although the latter is a lesser consideration with the "free" locally available databases.

In the reference interview, the librarian must ascertain the purpose of the search to tailor it to the user's needs or to advise the user as to which database(s) to search first for a particular topic. A search to find references for a clinical care rounds presentation should be handled differently from a search for a dissertation topic, grant proposal, research project, or term paper. The clinician may be satisfied with a few recent citations on the topic, whereas the researcher and doctoral candidate will prefer to have an exhaustive search processed over more than one database [13]. Cogswell points out that this individualized service is not generally found with more traditional manual literature search services. As a result, the service has led to an increased awareness by the user of the complexity of information retrieval and the high degree of specialization and knowledge required of reference librarians [14]. This awareness has been even further kindled by the presence of locally available databases that the user can search directly.

A primary advantage to using a bibliographic database versus its printed counterpart is the flexibility possible in accessing the various elements (any single component of the bibliographic unit record: author[s], keyword[s] or subject descriptors, journal, title, year, etc.) of the unit record. While printed indexing and abstracting services provide a variety of separate access points—author index, subject index, report number index, etc.—the computerized unit record can be accessed simultaneously by requesting one or more of these elements using Boolean logic.

Manipulating the system is only the beginning; good searching requires a real understanding of how the databases are constructed as well as the level of indexing provided by the database producer. It should also be noted that no single database covers all the literature in a field. Not only does the source coverage differ among databases, but indexing criteria and policies affect how thoroughly a source is indexed and whether a reference is retrieved. McCain et al. note, "In the 'real world' of online retrieval, the searcher is likely to employ an 'optimal' search strategy combining natural language and descriptors (or key citations) as the topic dictates" [15]. They conclude

> No single data base is likely to provide complete coverage of a complex, multidisciplinary literature. All data bases searched in this study provided relevant, novel documents.
> Citation retrieval should be considered an important adjunct to any descriptor-based searching. In certain queries, the citation data bases "outperformed" not only MEDLINE but EXCERPTA MEDICA and PSYCInfo as well [16].

The databases primarily used in health sciences libraries contain bibliographic data and have their counterparts in printed indexes and abstracts. There are, however, a growing number of databases that provide factual information but do not always have printed counterparts (e.g., CHEMLINE [CHEMical dictionary onLINE], Toxicology Data Bank [TDB]). These will be discussed briefly.

NLM DATABASES

The National Library of Medicine's MEDLINE database was one of the first online databases to appear for general use and remains the primary database used in health sciences libraries. Its printed counterparts include *Index Medicus, International Nursing Index,* and *Index to Dental Literature.*

5.1 *MEDLINE (MEDlars onLINE).* Bethesda, MD, National Library of Medicine.

The MEDLINE database covers the most recent three to four years of the medical journal literature from 1966 to the present, with BACKFILES for earlier references. Other vendors have a variety of chronological groupings of this database, including a single file covering all years. MEDLINE covers references to more than 3,738 journals as well as a small number of conference proceedings and chapters of multiauthored books from 1974 to 1982. The scope of the MEDLINE file is broad and includes basic life sciences material as well as medicine and allied health. The coverage is international, with one-third to one-half of the references to non-English-language articles.

The average article is indexed with approximately twelve MeSH descriptors, three to five of them are designated as the primary concepts discussed in the article. These primary subject descriptors are the subject headings under which the reference appears in the printed *Index Medicus* (or other index). However, all twelve are searchable on MEDLINE and include such frequently mentioned concepts as *age groups, gender, geographic areas, experimental animals*, and *humans*. These concepts are not generally listed in the printed *Index Medicus*. The searcher using MEDLINE, thus, can search not only major concepts of an article but also secondary concepts discussed in that article. The depth of indexing is one of the strong features of MEDLINE as a bibliographic source because the searcher need not rely on the title of an article alone to reveal the article's scope. Keyword/textword searching of specific terms from the titles and abstracts is possible as a way of refining a search on a very specific topic. The MEDLINE file includes author abstracts from the articles, when available, which are searchable, as opposed to only the citations available in the printed indexes represented in this database. While MEDLINE provides best value in searching the medical literature, a comprehensive search across databases such as Excerpta Medica's EMBASE, PsychInfo, and BIOSIS Previews will yield additional relevant references [17-18].

In addition to being available through NLM, MEDLINE is available from the major vendors. The full file or subsets have also been mounted locally by a number of academic health sciences centers for their clientele. The database is available from CD-ROM vendors for use with both IBM and Macintosh hardware.

5.2 *TOXLINE (TOXicology literature onLINE)*. Bethesda, MD, National Library of Medicine.

5.3 *CHEMLINE (CHEMical dictionary onLINE)*. Bethesda, MD, National Library of Medicine.

5.4 *CHEMID (CHEMical IDentification)*. Bethesda, MD, National Library of Medicine.

The TOXLINE databases provide access to references in the toxicological literature—journal articles, monographs, dissertations, published proceedings, etc.—from a number of bibliographic secondary sources and toxicology "research in progress" from the Computer Retrieval of Information on Scientific Projects (CRISP) files, the latter of which provide information on research projects for the current three years. The subfiles include references (some with abstracts) from Aneuploidy File; Environmental Mutagen Information Center File (EMIC); Environmental Teratology Information Center File (ETIC); Epidemiology Information System; Hazardous Materials Technical Center; International Labor Office; National Institute for Occupational Safety and Health Technical Information Center File; Pesticides Abstracts (PESTAB); Poisonous Plants Bibliography; Toxicity Bibliography; Toxicology Document and Data Depository; Toxicology Research Projects; Toxic Substances Control Act Test Submissions; Chemical-Biological Activities; International Pharmaceutical Abstracts (IPA); and Toxicological Aspects of Environmental Health [19]. The files are in four parts: TOXLINE, covering 1981-1992; TOXLINE65, covering pre-1965-1980; TOXLIT, covering 1981-1992; and TOXLIT65, covering 1965-1980. The TOXLIT files contain the information from the Chemical Abstracts Service and are updated monthly.

This file, unlike MEDLINE, is searched primarily with natural language terms (free text) from titles and abstracts. The use of synonyms is the primary search method, including right-hand truncation of root words, i.e., to retrieve terms beginning with "mutagen," a truncation symbol would follow the term to indicate that all possible suffixes are wanted. Thus, "mutagen#" would retrieve:

> mutagen
> mutagenicity
> mutagens, etc.

Logically this would be the equivalent of "OR"-ing these terms in a search statement. The Chemical Abstracts Service (CAS) registry numbers can be used to search the *CA, BA, IPA, PESTAB, EMIC,* and *ETIC* portions of the file. All MeSH descriptors cannot be used directly; however, "uniterms" (single words) from the MeSH vocabulary are searchable in the TOXBIB subfile. As with all textword searching, a large number of synonyms must be used to search effectively for type of organism, age, or sex concepts.

Citations retrieved include author, title, source journal, secondary source identifier (e.g., *CA* or *TOXBIB*), and abstracts. The file has not been edited for duplicates, so the same citation may be retrieved from more than one subfile [20].

CHEMLINE is a companion file to the TOXLINE files. As a chemical dictionary, CHEMLINE provides synonyms and CAS registry numbers (also searchable in MEDLINE) that aid in developing a search strategy. CHEMLINE, in addition to its uses as a dictionary file for TOXLINE and the TOXNET files, can also be searched as a data file for chemical information, including molecular formula and structure. In health sciences libraries, CHEMLINE is generally used in the preparation of a bibliographic search in TOXLINE or other free-text databases, rather than as a search for more technical chemical information.

The CHEMID database first appeared in 1990 as a chemical dictionary thesaurus that contains more than 267,000 chemical substances, cited by Registry Number (RN) in the following NLM databases: TOXLINE, TOXLINE65, TOXLIT, TOXLIT65, MEDLINE and its BACKFILES, MeSH, AIDSLINE, CANCERLIT, CCRIS, ETICBACK, HSDB, and RTECS. Some substances listed in CHEMID from RTECS do not have registry numbers. Both CHEMLINE and CHEMID are helpful in identifying terms and registry numbers, which can be used when cross-searching several databases for a substance.

5.5 *AIDSLINE (AIDS onLINE)*. Bethesda, MD, National Library of Medicine.
5.6 *CANCERLIT (CANCER LITerature)*. Bethesda, MD, National Library of Medicine. Formerly: *CANCERLINE*
5.7 *PDQ (Physician Data Query)*. Bethesda, MD, National Library of Medicine.

AIDSLINE became available on the ELHILL database in 1988 with records from MEDLINE, AIDS-related records from the HEALTH file in April 1989, and the CANCERLIT file in July 1989. The file currently has more than 81,000 records and is searched using *MeSH*. Records for AIDS-related meeting abstracts began being indexed in 1990, including the Fifth International Conference on AIDS held in Montreal in June 1989, the Symposium on Nonhuman Primate Models for AIDS, and the annual meeting of the American Society for Microbiology. A phased implementation of adding AIDS-related citations from other MEDLARS files is planned [21-22]. The file is updated weekly.

CANCERLIT, a component of the International Cancer Research Data Bank (ICRDB) Program, contains 350,000 references from *Carcinogenesis Abstracts* 1963-1976 and *Cancer Therapy Abstracts* (formerly *Cancer Chemotherapy Abstracts*) 1967-1980, as well as selected symposia reports, monographs, and proceedings since 1977. Searching is done primarily by using natural language terms from titles and abstracts. Abstracts in this file are lengthy and informative. As the sources of publications indicate, this file is most successful for searching topics related to carcinogenesis and cancer therapy, but not necessarily other cancer topics. Since 1976, however, the file has included all cancer topics, with all articles except case histories indexed from the primary cancer literature. This file is updated monthly and contains more than 965,000 records.

Specific topics with no *MeSH* equivalent, like MOPP or DAFT, two combination chemotherapy acronyms, are more successfully searched on the CANCERLIT file than on MEDLINE. Conversely, topics that are broad or have many synonyms, e.g., embryonal and experimental tumors, may be more successfully searched on MEDLINE. In addition to the standard bibliographic information, citations include the abstracts and author address (useful for verifying a particular author with a common name and for obtaining reprint addresses) [23].

The PDQ database (also from the ICRDB program), on the other hand, is designed to provide state-of-the-art information on cancer therapy and cancer clinical trials for physicians and their patients. Details of the specific protocols have been deleted and only the general information on the protocol objectives and patient entry criteria are described for 700 NCI supported protocols. Names, addresses, and telephone numbers of contact people at each participating institution are also given. Free text and index term searching are used. The file is updated monthly.

5.8 *HEALTH PLANNING AND ADMIN (HEALTH PLANNING AND ADMINistration)*. Bethesda, MD, National Library of Medicine.
5.9 *BIOETHICSLINE (BIOETHICS onLINE)*. Bethesda, MD, National Library of Medicine.
5.10 *HISTLINE (HISTory of medicine onLINE)*. Bethesda, MD, National Library of Medicine.
5.11 *POPLINE (POPulation information onLINE)*. Bethesda, MD, National Library of Medicine.

The HEALTH file, available since the fall of 1978, is produced in cooperation with the American Hospital Association and the National Library of Medicine. It contains more than 680,000 references to worldwide literature in the fields of health planning and administration (organization, workforce, financing, etc.), and health care delivery. The initial file contains references from MEDLINE, *Hospital Literature Index*, and selected journals emphasizing health care. Journal coverage of HEALTH is listed in the annual *List of Serials Indexed for Online Users* published by NLM and distributed through the National Technical Information Services (NTIS). The file is updated monthly. Searching primarily uses MeSH vocabulary. The HEALTH file has the advantage over MEDLINE of covering references back to 1975 in a single file, although there is a great deal of overlap between HEALTH and MEDLINE for "current" MEDLINE years. Citations are available with abstracts in some instances. This file, like MEDLINE, is available on CD-ROM and through the major database vendors.

BIOETHICSLINE is a cross-disciplinary file of more than 38,600 references to both print and nonprint material indexed since 1973 for the *Bibliography of Bioethics*, developed by the Center for Bioethics, Kennedy Institute of Ethics, Georgetown University. Included are references to journal and newspaper articles, books, court decisions, bills, state and federal statutes, and audiovisual materials. This database provides the most interdisciplinary material of any of the NLM databases. It includes references from the literature of law, religion, psychology, philosophy, the popular media, as well as the health sciences. All references are to English-language sources. While computer mapping is done to link BIOETHICS keywords to

MeSH terms, searching is best done using a combination of *MeSH*, terms from the *BIOETHICS Thesaurus*, or textwords from the title.

HISTLINE contains more than 110,500 references for the NLM *Bibliography of the History of Medicine*. Included are references to journal articles, monographs, and symposia in the history of medicine from 1970 to the present, with selected references back to 1964. Updating is quarterly, with approximately 4,500 citations added per year. The file is international in scope and is searched using a special vocabulary based on *MeSH*. NLM is planning to make this file available at no charge as a part of the NLM Locator, the Library's INTERNET catalog, in the near future.

The POPLINE database covers the literature of family planning, fertility control, population, and reproduction. The original database, POPIN-FORM, consisted of a file maintained since 1973 by the Population Information Program (PIP) of Johns Hopkins University and the Center for Population and Family Health Library/Information Program of Columbia University. It is currently maintained by PIP with the assistance of *Population Index* at Princeton University. Most citations date from 1970; however, there are selected references that date back to 1886. The current file consists of citations with abstracts for a variety of materials including journal articles, monographs, and technical reports. Updated monthly, the database contains more than 199,900 citations and increases annually by approximately 10,000 records. MeSH terms or keywords from the *POPLINE Thesaurus* can be used for searching. Textword searching of titles and abstracts is also possible.

The scope of the database has recently been changed and new selection criteria developed. All print formats are represented, "including: journal articles, monographs, monograph chapters, conference papers, wall charts, technical reports, procedure manuals, press releases, contractor submissions, working papers, bills, laws, court decisions, patents, training manuals, theses, and conference proceedings, as well as annual reports, pamphlets, and newspaper articles" [24].

5.12 *AIDSTRIALS*. Bethesda, MD, National Library of Medicine.
5.13 *AIDSDRUGS*. Bethesda, MD, National Library of Medicine.
5.14 *BIOTECHSEEK*. Bethesda, MD, National Library of Medicine.
5.15 *DENTALPROJ*. Bethesda, MD, National Library of Medicine.

AIDSTRIALS and AIDSDRUGS were introduced in 1989 as factual databases. AIDSTRIALS provides information on clinical trials of agents being evaluated for their effectiveness against Acquired Immunodeficiency Syndrome (AIDS), HIV infections, and AIDS-related diseases. Records include information on

1. Name of the trial.
2. Purpose or summary of the trial.
3. Agent(s) being studied.
4. Patient eligibility criteria.
5. Status of the trial (open or closed to new patients).
6. Location where the study is being conducted.

Information on the more than 400 trials listed in the database is from the National Institute of Allergy and Infectious Diseases (NIAID), National Institutes of Health (NIH), and the Food and Drug Administration (FDA).

AIDSDRUGS serves as a companion database to AIDSTRIALS, providing specific information on the agents (190 as of Nov. 1993) being tested in clinical trials. Although primarily a factual database, up to ten bibliographic references are listed in the record for each agent [25-26].

BIOTECHSEEK, also known as BIOSEEK, was introduced in 1990 and indexes approximately thirty biotechnology journals not indexed for MEDLINE. Subject searching uses the MeSH vocabulary and the database is structured like MEDLINE. The database contains more than 3,500 records.

The DENTALPROJ database contains information on research projects supported by the National Institute of Dental Research since 1989. In March 1990, records for research projects from the Department of Defense were added. In all, there are only 786 projects listed through May 1992. Searching is done using *MeSH* and keywords [27].

A separate computer system operates the Toxicology Data Network (TOXNET) databases at NLM. These files include:

5.16 *Chemical Carcinogenesis Research Information System (CCRIS).* Bethesda, MD, National Library of Medicine.

5.17 *Developmental and Reproductive Toxicology (DART).* Bethesda, MD, National Library of Medicine.

5.18 *GENE-TOX (Genetic Toxicology Program File).* Bethesda, MD, National Library of Medicine.

The CCRIS database is sponsored by the National Cancer Institute and provides information on chemicals thought to be carcinogenic. CCRIS has its own vocabulary that has online explanations to guide a searcher to the proper term for a particular concept, e.g., the term used for a particular species found in the CCRIS database. The file is small, with a little more than 4,400 records.

The DART database is a bibliographic database of references to the literature on agents that cause birth defects. It is supported by the National Institute of Environmental Health Sciences, the Environmental Protection Agency, the Agency of Toxic Substances and Disease Registry, and the

National Library of Medicine. The bibliographic citations are indexed using the MeSH vocabulary and CAS Registry Numbers (RN), which are fully searchable.

DART is the continuation of the Environmental Teratology Information Center Backfile (ETICBACK), which covers the literature from 1950-1988. About 60% of the DART file comes from MEDLINE, while the remaining 40% of the file includes citations for abstracts of meetings, symposia proceedings, monographs, technical reports, and articles from non-MEDLINE journals [28]. MeSH indexing is supplemented by additional chemical indexing in this file.

The backfile of the Environmental Mutagen, Carcinogen and Teratogen Information Program of the Oak Ridge National Laboratory (EMICBACK) covers the literature from 1950-1988 for agents that have been tested for genotoxic activity [29] and, like ETICBACK, is on the TOXNET computer. Both EMICBACK and ETICBACK are also available as subsets of TOXLINE on ELHILL.

The GENE-TOX database, created by the U.S. Environmental Protection Agency (EPA), was introduced in 1991 and contains genetic toxicology data on more than 2,900 chemicals. The data have been peer reviewed and referenced. In addition to Substance Identification (ID) information and Chemical Classification Category (CCAT), records contain an EMIC/EMICBACK reference number and panel report citation to the official report that evaluated the specific test system. Cross-file searching with CCRIS (5.16) and RTECS (5.20) is also possible [30].

5.19 *Hazardous Substance Data Bank (HSDB)*. Bethesda, MD, National Library of Medicine.

5.20 *Registry of Toxic Effects of Chemical Substances (RTECS)*. Bethesda, MD, National Library of Medicine.

5.21 *Integrated Risk Information System (IRIS)*. Bethesda, MD, National Library of Medicine.

5.22 *Toxic Chemical Release Inventory (TRI)*. Bethesda, MD, National Library of Medicine.

HSDB is a factual (nonbibliographic) database that provides information on more than 4,300 hazardous chemicals. Information on emergency medical treatment, safety and handling, environmental fate, exposure potential, and regulatory requirements are included for each record. The information is peer reviewed by toxicologists and other experts.

The RTECS file, another factual database, contains information on the toxic effects of more than 120,000 chemicals. Created by the National Institute of Occupational Health and Safety, records include data on skin/eye irritation, carcinogenicity, mutagenicity, and reproductive effects.

The IRIS database, sponsored by the EPA, contains information on the health risks of more than 600 chemicals. EPA Health Advisories from the Office of Drinking Water and information on environmental standards and regulations are also included.

The TRI files, of which there are now four (TRI87, TRI88, TRI89, TRI90), provide information collected from industry on estimated release of toxic chemicals to the environment (air, water, land, and underground injection) that have been mandated by the Emergency Planning and Community Right-to-Know Act. These data are compiled annually [31]. TRIFACTS, a companion file, became available in Spring 1992 and provides nontechnical information on the TRI chemicals using nontechnical language, whereas the TRI, HSDB, and IRIS scientific language may be too difficult to understand [32].

Cross-file searching on commonly indexed elements, e.g., CAS Registry Numbers in TOXNET files, makes searching for a particular agent efficient among the TOXNET files.

NON-NLM DATABASES

5.23 *BIOSIS Previews*. Philadelphia, PA, BioSciences Information Service.

The BIOSIS Previews database contains references to literature in periodicals, monographs, dissertations, published proceedings, translation journals, nomenclature rules, and other sources indexed for *Biological Abstracts (BA)* and *Biological Abstracts/RRM* (formerly *Bioresearch Index— BIORI*) since 1969. Journal coverage overlap with MEDLINE is 84%, with the "medically oriented" references representing 82% of the file from 1981-1985 [33]. Each citation includes the bibliographic reference: *BA* or *BA/RRM* abstract number; journal coden (a five-letter code for the title); subject descriptors provided by BIOSIS indexers; primary, secondary, and tertiary subject concept codes (numerical codes used to index broad subject areas in biology. For example, "neoplasms" and "neoplastic agents—diagnostic methods" as a concept could be searched using the concept code CC24001); and biosystematic codes representing taxonomic groups of organisms discussed in the article. A language field, added in January 1978, allows for the limiting of retrieval to specific languages. Searching can also be done using natural language words from the titles, keywords assigned by BIOSIS indexers, authors' names, numerical codes for broad subject categories (concept codes), and taxonomic codes (biosystematic codes).

Searching the BIOSIS database is much easier than searching the printed indexes in *BA* and *BA/RRM*. Use of the biosystematic and concept codes facilitates searching of broad topics and eliminates having to use numerous synonyms, as contrasted to an awkward, laborious search using the concept codes or the biosystematic codes in the printed indexes. Indexer-assigned keywords augment terms from the titles with both common names of animals as well as genus and species names for animals that are not mentioned in the title of an article. Many words are segmented to add further flexibility to searching, e.g., adreno cortical, neuro physiology, pseudo protein.

Searching BIOSIS Previews can provide complementary references to a MEDLINE search for the book, meeting, and report literature [34-35]. In a recent study, Brandsma et al. found "overlap between the files occurs less than 50% of the time" [36].

5.24 *CA Search*. Columbus, OH, Chemical Abstracts Service.

CA Search provides online access to more than 14,000 journals, monographs, dissertations, conference reports, patents, technical reports, and reviews indexed for *Chemical Abstracts (CA)* from 1970 to the present. Keyword indexes from the biweekly issues of *CA* and *CASIA (CA Subject Index Alert)* controlled vocabulary of the volume indexes are included.

The unit record does not include an abstract but does include the *CA* abstract number, complete bibliographic information, journal coden, language, publication type, and keyword phrases from the biweekly issue of *CA* and the *CA* section where the citation appeared.

Searching is primarily by use of natural language terms from titles and keywords (and abbreviations in keywords) added by indexers; *CA* subject sections, authors' names, language, and type of publication are also searchable. The CAS Registry Number, an essential identifier in searching for a specific substance, is not a searchable element in all vendors' systems. This should be kept in mind when choosing a vendor for *CA* searching. STN International provides the most comprehensive searching of *CA*, including structure and formula searching options.

5.25 *CINAHL*. Glendale, CA, Glendale Adventists Medical Center.

The CINAHL database provides access to the *Cumulative Index to Nursing and Allied Health Literature* from 1983 to date. The database includes abstracts from more than 150 journals that are regularly indexed. CINAHL subject headings, similar to *MeSH*, are used for subject searching. Online access is available via BRS, Data-Star, and DIALOG. It is also available on CD-ROM from several vendors, as well as on tape from the producer.

5.26 *EMBASE (Excerpta Medica dataBASE).* Amsterdam and Princeton, NJ, Excerpta Medica.

EMBASE became available from DIALOG in 1978. The file includes references from all the sections of *Excerpta Medica*. References to articles from 4,500 journals (3,500 regularly indexed) comprise 95% of the database, with references from monographs and dissertations comprising the remaining 5% of the file. The database is limited to human medicine and related basic sciences. There are some references to allied health, dentistry, nursing, psychology, and veterinary medicine in the database; they are not specifically included, and specialty journals in these fields are not indexed.

Unit records in EMBASE contain the citation number, which does not correspond to an abstract number in the printed *EM;* the bibliographic citation; *Excerpta Medica* classification numbers, EMCLAS, for all the sections in which the citation was printed; the indexing terms from the *EMTREE Thesaurus;* natural language terms; EMTAGS, frequently mentioned concepts such as "review articles," "fetus," "embryo," etc. [37]; and the abstract. In January 1979, EMBASE records began containing references to the printed journal. A record listed for more than one EM section refers to the abstract number in the most relevant section for that reference.

Searching is done using a combination of free text and terms from the *EMTREE Thesaurus,* with author searching, EMCLAS, and EMTAG searching also possible. The current *EMTREE Thesaurus* (3d ed. 1992) contains 35,000 medical and drug terms in two volumes. Volume 1 includes a tree structure and volume 2 includes an alphabetical index, EMCLAS, EMTAGS, LINKS, and an EMBASE user manual.

EMBASE represents the entire *Excerpta Medica* file, whereas the printed sections contain only 60% of the online file. This variation is due in part to the editorial policies of *Excerpta Medica,* which allow each section editor to determine whether citations included in that section are to be included in the printed journal section or remain only available online. Therefore, 40% of the records in the *Excerpta Medica* files are never listed in the printed sections and are only available online.

In deciding whether to search MEDLINE or EMBASE, one should keep in mind the needs of users and the primary content of the two databases. MEDLINE contains a large number of U.S. journals, such as state medical journals and NIH Consensus Development Conference Summaries; EMBASE has more foreign journal coverage. As to vocabulary, MEDLINE uses American English spelling of terms, while EMBASE uses somewhat different British/European spelling and vocabulary. Subheading access on MEDLINE versus EMTAG access on EMBASE should also be considered. On the other hand, some bound terms in MEDLINE, such as "CHROMO-

SOMES, G-12" are awkward to use; whereas with EMBASE the specific chromosome number is easily searchable.

5.27 *EPILEPSYLINE (EPILEPSY onLINE)*. Bethesda, MD, National Institute of Neurological and Communicative Disorders and Stroke.

EPILEPSYLINE, sponsored by the National Institute of Neurological and Communicative Disorders and Stroke (NINCDS), is available through DIALOG. The citations are obtained from Excerpta Medica's *Epilepsy Abstracts* as well as additional material on the experimental aspects of seizures and convulsions. The database is international in scope, covering literature from 1945 to the present, and is updated monthly. Subject searching is through textwords from titles and abstracts as well as Excerpta Medica's MALIMET vocabulary and classification codes found in the *EMBASE Thesaurus Guide*.

5.28 *PsychInfo*. Lancaster, PA, American Psychological Association.

Corresponding to the printed version of *Psychological Abstracts* from 1967 to date, the database contains references to articles from more than 800 journals, as well as from monographs, dissertations, technical reports, and conference reports. Each unit record includes the *Psychological Abstracts* abstract number, bibliographic information including author's address, language, year of publication, subject descriptors from the *Thesaurus of Psychological Index Terms* (Arlington, VA: American Psychological Association, 1991), abstract, and subject index phrases from the volume and cumulative indexes of *Psychological Abstracts*.

A combination of searching thesaurus terms and natural language terms from titles and abstracts is most successful. Now in its sixth edition since 1973, the *Thesaurus of Psychological Index Terms* has evolved into a useful tool to facilitate searching. The relationship section (main listing) provides detailed information about each thesaurus term. A rotated alphabetical terms section, similar to a permuted index, lists each word and all terms in which it appears. In addition there is a cluster section, which arranges the terms into eight broad categories (disorders cluster, educational cluster, geographical cluster, legal cluster, occupational and employment cluster, statistical cluster, tests and testing cluster, treatment cluster) which are in turn each divided into a number of subsections. There are three appendices: new postable terms; new nonpostable terms, cross-references; and content classification categories and codes.

Searching prior to 1973, before the *Thesaurus* was fully developed, is more successful using free-text terms. Language, publication type, year of publication, and author are also searchable fields. In addition, specific psychological tests are searchable. A topic such as the psychological aspects of abortion could be searched appropriately on MEDLINE, EMBASE, and the PsychInfo file.

5.29 *SCISEARCH.* Philadelphia, PA, Institute for Scientific Information.

SCISEARCH is a multidisciplinary database indexing the literature of science and technology. Records correspond to the published *Science Citation Index (SCI)* with additional citations from the *Current Contents* series not included in *SCI.* The database covers January 1974 to date and includes all significant references (articles, reports of meetings, letters, editorials, correction notices, etc.) from 3,700 scientific and technical journals. Subject coverage in the life and health sciences is roughly divided as follows: life sciences, 23%; clinical practice, 12%; and agriculture, biology, and environmental sciences, 11%. The remainder of the database is composed of citations in the physical sciences and technology. In 1988, research fronts were added to the database.

In addition to the bibliographic record, citations give information on language, author's address, and number of references, including all cited references. Searching this file has some special capabilities due to the unique feature of the file's records. Retrieval can be by natural language terms from the title and author address fields. In the Citation Index (comprising references from the bibliographies of Source Index citations), the following elements are directly searchable: name of first author, journal title, volume number, first page of the item, year of publication, and code for the type of publication. In 1988, titles of cited articles became both searchable and displayable.

The searchable fields in the Source Index include names of all authors, addresses of all authors (where given), title in English, actual title (if not in English), journal title, volume and issue numbers, inclusive pagination of the item, year of publication, code for type of publication, number of references, and Institute for Scientific Information (ISI) journal issue accession number. Beginning in 1991, source articles began appearing with English-language abstracts and accompany about 50% of the references, including 44% of the references from non-English-language sources [38]. Also in 1991, additional indexing terms were added to augment the terms from titles [39].

Citation Index searching can be valuable when it is known that relevant material on a topic will be scattered through more than one discipline or buried in the text of a seemingly nonrelevant paper, e.g., a specific method or technique with varied applications. Citations begin to appear from nine to twelve months after the original article appears in print, so very recent articles will not be useful for citation searching. The multidisciplinary subject coverage of this file is also a useful feature for some search topics. Another helpful feature of the file is the one- to three-week time lag between publication and entry into the file. This continues to be the case even with the inclusion of additional indexing and abstracts. Snow's study reveals, "SCISEARCH proved to be at least one issue ahead of other health sciences files in indexing 19 out of 30 titles...In the remaining 37% of the sample, both MEDLINE and SCISEARCH offered equally-timely coverage" [40].

Citation searching does have pitfalls along with its usefulness. For example, searching a cited author's name such as Harris TB, will (1) retrieve all earlier papers written by Harris in any subject on any aspect of Harris research that was cited; (2) retrieve papers because they cited Harris working in another field of research; (3) retrieve all papers citing earlier works by Harris TB, even though some were by Thomas B., by Teresa B., and yet others by T. Bradford; (4) fail to retrieve articles that cited relevant papers by Harris when Harris was not the first author; and (5) fail to retrieve articles that cited relevant papers by Harris because Harris' first initial was not used in the reference or because the initials were inverted.

5.30 *IPA (International Pharmaceutical Abstracts)*. Bethesda, MD, American Society of Hospital Pharmacists.

IPA indexes and abstracts articles from the worldwide pharmaceutical literature. The database contains literature in three broad categories. Fifty percent of it deals with drug actions, toxicity, drug evaluations, drug interaction, etc. Thirty percent of the literature is in the area of research—biopharmaceutics, pharmaceuticals, drug stability, pharmacology, pharmaceutical chemistry, drug analysis, pharmacognosy, and methodology. The remaining 20% deals with pharmaceutical technology; pharmacy practice; legislation, laws, and regulations; economics, etc. In addition to the bibliographic reference, records contain as many as ten index terms, and numerous cross-references to trade names, chemical names, investigational drug numbers, and concepts. CAS registry numbers are also searchable. The database includes more than 750,000 records from 1970 to the present and adds approximately 7,000 citations a year with monthly updates.

SELECTIVE DISSEMINATION OF INFORMATION SEARCHES

Selective Dissemination of Information (SDI) searches are available from BRS, DIALOG, and NLM for some of their files. With this service, search profiles are stored in the computer and automatically processed against each file update, usually on a monthly basis. For the files discussed in this chapter, BRS provides monthly SDI capabilities for BIOSIS Previews,

MEDLINE, PsychInfo, and CA Search; DIALOG provides monthly SDI service for MEDLINE, TOXLINE, and CANCERLIT on a monthly basis. There are also commercial SDI services such as the Automatic Subject Citation Alert (ASCA) service offered by the Institute for Scientific Information.

> 5.31 *CURRENT CONTENTS SEARCH.* Philadelphia, PA, Institute for Scientific Information.
> 5.32 *REFERENCE UPDATE.* Carlsbad, CA, Research Information Systems.
> 5.33 *EMBASE Selects.* New York, Elsevier Scientific Publishers, Electronic Publishing Division.

The current two years of *Current Contents* references are available online via BRS and DIALOG as CURRENT CONTENTS SEARCH. The *Current Contents* sections (*see* 4.18-4.21) are available for subscription on diskette with weekly updates, with or without abstracts.

REFERENCE UPDATE is another current awareness tool that became available in 1988 on disk. The basic service provides reference to 400 "core" journals in the life sciences, while the deluxe edition covers 1,100 journals. There is also a monthly *Clinical Edition* for Internal Medicine and a *Meetings Edition* that provides references to the proceedings of well-known societies such as FASEB, the Society for Neuroscience, the Biophysical Society, and the International Association for Dental Research. Abstracts are available online through Research Information Systems' Abstract *Express* service.

Both CURRENT CONTENTS and REFERENCE UPDATE are available in IBM, Macintosh, and NEC 9800 Series versions.

Elsevier has recently introduced a current alerting service, EMBASE Selects, on a subscription basis with weekly updates on disk, tape, or cassette formats. Subscribers may custom select from a list of 3,500 journals indexed in EMBASE. References include the standard bibliographic information with abstract in ASCII format [41].

DATABASE SOURCES

There are many other databases that have relevance to the health sciences. The following sources provide more exhaustive lists of available databases, providing information on database producers, vendors (e.g., BRS, DIALOG), and distributors (e.g., CD-ROM and disk licensers).

Computer-readable Data Bases: a directory and data source book. Martha E. Williams, editor-in-chief. Chicago, American Library Association, 1985.

DataBase Directory. White Plains, NY, Knowledge Industry. In cooperation with the American Society for Information Science, 1984- . Semiannual, Fall 1985- . Annual, 1984/85.
Directory of Online Healthcare Databases. Oak Park, IL, Albine Guild. 1985- . [Annual?].
Fulltext Sources Online. Needham Heights, MA, BiblioData. 1989- . Semiannual. Each new edition supersedes all previous editions.
Gale Directory of Databases. Kathleen Young Marcaccio, ed. Detroit, MI, Gale, 1993- . Formed by the merger of *Gale's Computer-readable Databases* and Cuadra/Gale's *Directory of Online Databases* and *Directory of Portable Databases.*

Successful searching requires constant awareness of database and vendor system changes. The vendors provide monthly newsletters to subscribers, which contain information on system changes and database updates. In addition, the database producers provide information on changes in their files, vocabularies, etc.

Other opportunities for keeping up-to-date on searching are provided through workshops connected with library schools' continuing education programs, regional and local users' groups, and programs at regional and national meetings of organizations such as the Medical Library Association, as well as workshops offered by database producers and vendors. The journal literature regularly provides articles on searching techniques and databases. *Medical Reference Services Quarterly* has a regular column on searching, as does *Library Journal.* Journals devoted to electronic formats include *Online, Online Review, Database Searcher,* and *CD-ROM Review.* These journals regularly have articles on searching specific databases and comparison of databases for searching specific subject areas, which can be quite useful in keeping up with changes and new features of the databases.

Each library and its clientele will determine which files will be most useful for that library to offer. However, the use of electronic databases as primary reference tools has become so essential that all provisions should be made to ensure that the reference collection includes availability to the most pertinent databases (either online, locally mounted, or from portable formats) for the library's clientele, and that the staff maintains its expertise in as many search methods as possible.

REFERENCES

1. Lancaster FW. Whither libraries? or wither libraries. Coll Res Lib 1978 Sept;39:356.

2. McCarn DB, Leiter J. Online services in medicine and beyond. Science 1973 July 27;181:218-24.

3. Author's survey, Fall 1991. (unpublished)

4. Werner G. Use of online bibliographic retrieval services in health sciences libraries in the United States and Canada. Bull Med Libr Assoc 1979 Jan;67:1-14.

5. Werner, Use of online retrieval, 1-14.

6. Author's survey, Fall 1991. (unpublished)

7. Morris RT, Holtum EA, Curry DS. Being there: the effect of the user's presence on MEDLINE search results. Bull Med Libr Assoc 1982 July;70:298-304.

8. Salomon K, Burgess C. Patron presence during the online search: attitudes of university librarians. Online Rev 1984;8(6):549-58.

9. Ibid.

10. Salomon, Patron presence, 554.

11. Somerville AN. The place of the reference interview in computer searching: the academic setting. Online 1977 Oct;1:12-23.

12. Somerville AN. The pre-search reference interview—a step by step guide. Database 1982 Feb;5:32-38.

13. Wagner J. Multiple database use. Online 1977 Jan;1:35-41.

14. Cogswell JS. Online search services: implications for libraries and library users. Coll Res Lib 1978 July;39:275-80.

15. McCain KW, White HD, Griffith BC. Comparing retrieval performances in online data bases. Info Proc Manag 1987;23(6):552.

16. Ibid.

17. Ibid.

18. Brandsma R, Deurenberg-Vos HWH, Bakker S, Brand-de-Heer DL, Otten RHJ, Pinatsas A. A comparison of the coverage of clinical medicine provided by BIOSIS Previews and MEDLINE. Online Rev 1990;14(6):367-75.

19. Wexler P. The framework of toxicology information. Toxicology 1990 Jan-Feb;60(1-2):76.

20. Schutheisz RJ. TOXLINE: evolution of an online interactive bibliographic database. J Am Soc Info Sci 1981 Nov;34:421-29.

21. AIDSLINE Update. NLM Tech Bull 1990 Feb;250:22.

22. AIDSLINE Update. NLM Tech Bull 1992 Jan-Feb;264:40-3.

23. Farmer J, Guillaumin B, Sorrentino S. CANCERLIT: a new look. NLM Tech Bull 1978 May;109:5-7.

24. POPLINE Update. NLM Tech Bull 1992 Jan-Feb;265:55.

25. AIDSTRIALS and AIDSDRUGS. NLM Tech Bull 1990 Feb;250:25.

26. See also: Dutcher GA. AIDSTRIALS and AIDSDRUGS. NLM Tech Bull 1989 July;243:17-27.

27. See: Bronson RJ. DENTALPROJ: an oral medicine database. Med Ref Serv Q 1990 Winter;9(4):81-91.

28. Arnesen SJ. Announcing a new bibliographic database on developmental reproductive toxicology: DART. NLM Tech Bull 1990 Apr;252:12-17.

29. Arensen SJ. EMICBACK: a new bibliographic database on TOXNET. NLM Tech Bull 1989 June;242:17-9.

30. Stroup D. GENE-TOX on TOXNET. NLM Tech Bull 1991 Mar-Apr;259:1,7-9.

31. TOXicology Data NETwork: a brief guide to searching its files. Bethesda, MD, Specialized Information Services. National Library of Medicine, 1991.

32. See Wexler P. TRIFACTS-a new TOXNET file. NLM Tech Bull May-June 1992;262:1,5-10.

33. Bruce NG, Farren AL. Searching BIOSIS Previews in the health care setting. Med Ref Serv Q 1987 Summer;6:17-27.

34. Ibid.

35. Brandsma et al. A comparison, 367-75.

36. Ibid., 371.

37. Guide to the classification and indexing system. Amsterdam/Princeton, NJ, Excerpta Medica, 1988; Appendix II:2.

38. Snow B. SCISEARCH changes: abstracts and added indexing. Online 1991 Sept;15:102-06.

39. Ibid.

40. Snow, SCISEARCH, 106.

41. EMBASE Selects, a new customized EMSCOPES Service. Info Today 1993 Sept; 10:4.

READINGS

Quint B. Inside a searcher's mind: the seven stages of an online search—part 1. Online 1991;15(3):13-8; part 2 Online 1991; 15(5):28-35.

Tenopir C. Issues in online database searching. Englewood CO: Libraries Unlimited, 1989. (Database Searching Series, no. 1.)

CHAPTER 6

U.S. Government Documents and Technical Reports

Fred W. Roper

U.S. GOVERNMENT DOCUMENTS

Government documents offer great potential as reference and information sources for health sciences libraries. Most topics of interest to researchers and practitioners in the health sciences are treated to some degree somewhere in a government publication. Unfortunately, these sources have the reputation of being difficult to work with. This perception derives from a lack of understanding both our government's organizational structure and the bibliographic tools that provide access to the publications. Consequently, U.S. government documents are often underused.

Government documents appear in print and nonprint formats; they are the materials that have been issued by the authority of a government, even if the government has not borne the expense of printing the publications. Although there are many printing offices connected with the various government agencies, the Government Printing Office (GPO) is the major supplier of U.S. government documents. The GPO does not print the majority of publications, but it does serve as the major distribution source for publications coming from the various agencies. The National Technical Information Service (NTIS) (discussed in the "Technical Reports" section) is another major distribution center for U.S. government documents.

Government publications are divided into three groups that roughly correspond to the three branches of government. *Congressional* publications relate to the work or proceedings of Congress, printed by the order, or for the use of, either the Senate or the House of Representatives. Court decisions published by the United States make up the bulk of *judicial* publications. *Executive* publications are published by the departments or the independent agencies of the executive branch of the government.

Libraries that request and qualify for depository library status can select the categories of publications most appropriate for their collections. Academic health sciences libraries are often associated with institutions whose main libraries have depository status and may receive depository materials in the health sciences on that basis. Libraries without depository status must select and acquire government publications from the GPO or other distribution outlets.

A major problem in dealing with government documents is the frequent changes that take place in government organizations. As agencies are abolished, created, or merged, their publications may also change. Organizational changes result in variations in bibliographic entry, which create difficulties for the librarian in locating the publications in appropriate catalogs and indexes. The secret of successful reference use of government documents lies largely in mastering the bibliographic sources that list them and in keeping up with organizational changes.

6.1 *Monthly Catalog of United States Government Publications.* Washington, DC, U.S. Government Printing Office, 1895- . Monthly; annual cumulative indexes.

The primary bibliography of U.S. government publications is the *Monthly Catalog of United States Government Publications,* which has been issued by the Superintendent of Documents since 1895. The *Catalog of Public Documents* was the primary index of documents until it ceased publication in 1940. Since that time, the *Monthly Catalog* has become increasingly more comprehensive, and improved indexes have made it easier to use.

In 1974, the Library Division of the Superintendent of Documents Office joined OCLC's online cataloging network, converted to the MARC format, and began cataloging according to Anglo-American Cataloging Rules (AACR). In 1976, citations in the *Monthly Catalog* appeared in a new format which made it a considerably improved source for cataloging information.

The basic arrangement of the entries in the *Monthly Catalog* is by Superintendent of Documents Classification Scheme. This arrangement is typically by agency because of the interdependence of the scheme with the organization of the federal government. Author, title, subject, and series/report indexes provide additional access to the documents. Cumulative indexes are published annually.

The current issues of the *Monthly Catalog* serve as both a catalog of documents coming to the attention of the Superintendent of Documents and an acquisitions source. Prices are given for the documents, but the actual cost may vary, due to changes after the catalog was published. These documents can be ordered from the GPO or from one of the other distribution sources indicated. A CD-ROM version of the *Monthly Catalog* is distributed by SilverPlatter and online access is available through BRS and DIALOG.

In addition to the general listing of government documents contained in the *Monthly Catalog,* individual agencies and departments may publish their own bibliographies and catalogs. These catalogs should be consulted for specific items published by a government unit.

> 6.2 *MEDOC: A Computerized Index to U.S. Government Documents in the Medical and Health Sciences.* Salt Lake City, UT, Eccles Health Sciences Library, University of Utah, 1974- . Quarterly, each issue cumulates; annual cumulation.

MEDOC is published quarterly with the final issue serving as a cumulation for the year. It is a computerized index of U.S. government publications considered to be important to health sciences libraries. MEDOC is prepared by the staff of the Spencer S. Eccles Health Sciences Library at the University of Utah, a depository library, and reflects the holdings of that library's documents collection.

The basic arrangement is by the Superintendent of Documents Classification Scheme with title/series, author, subject, and report number indexes. MeSH descriptors are used to create the subject index. MEDOC is available online through BRS.

TECHNICAL REPORTS

Health sciences librarians generally use technical reports less often than other types of materials. Reports are not easy to work with or locate and may be difficult to identify properly in some instances. To use technical reports effectively, librarians must become familiar with both the reference sources that maintain bibliographic control of reports and the primary acquisition and distribution centers.

Technical reports have achieved the potential for greater use in health sciences research with their increased availability through distribution centers and improved computer technologies. Since World War II, technical reports, like other types of materials in the sciences, have been used more frequently as a vehicle of communication. In the early period of extensive use, technical reports were considered only one step in the process of publication of a journal article or chapter in a monograph. Today they are often considered the final step in the publication process, although portions of many reports appear eventually in more formal literature. Their frequent citation in bibliographies and reading lists is evidence of increasing use;

librarians must be prepared to respond to growing pressure to verify and locate the cited reports.

A technical report normally is prepared for the agency for whom an investigation has been carried out. In general, a technical report either gives progress of the investigation currently being carried out or indicates the results of a completed investigation. The duration of the research project will determine the necessity for continuing progress reports or for one final report that covers all stages of the investigation. Quality of the content of technical reports tends to vary, because there is usually little, if any, quality control present in the form of refereeing. Material submitted to a journal, for example, undergoes much closer scrutiny than that in a technical report. However, the lack of restrictions on length and amount of material which can be included means the researcher might obtain considerably greater detail from a technical report than that found in a journal article.

Tallman [1] has characterized technical reports in the following manner.

1. There are many titles being published from a great many different agencies and organizations. Although there are not many distributing agencies, there is still enough complexity and variance to cause confusion.
2. There is a great range of quality in both form and content of the reports, ranging "from poorly written, brief, minor items of ephemeral value, to near print, well-organized, and comprehensive reports of relatively permanent value."
3. Distribution is often limited and may be based on an established need to have access to the material contained in the report.
4. The reports are not available from the usual book trade sources; they normally have to be obtained from special distribution centers.
5. Bibliographic control of technical reports has been confined, for the most part, to specialized sources; more conventional sources usually ignore them.
6. No union list exists of individual library holdings.
7. Handling is difficult once the reports are acquired because they may have multiple personal authors, several different identification numbers assigned to them, and formats that require binding or reinforcement for library use.
8. In many instances, the data contained in reports may be of great value to the public and may be the only detailed source of information available on the topic.

The major collection and distribution centers for technical reports in the United States are government agencies: National Technical Information Service (NTIS), National Aeronautics and Space Administration (NASA),

Department of Energy (DOE), and Educational Resources Information Center (ERIC). The principal collection and distribution center in the United Kingdom is the British Library Document Supply Centre (BLDSC).

National Technical Information Service

Established in 1945 as the Publication Board in the U.S. Department of Commerce, NTIS has successively been known as the Office of Technical Services, the Clearinghouse for Federal Scientific and Technical Information, and the National Technical Information Service. Although its scope has changed with its name changes, the center's basic purpose of supplying copies of unclassified government technical reports has remained. Today NTIS serves as the "central source for public sale of government-sponsored research and development reports and other analyses prepared by Federal agencies, their contractors and grantees" [2]. The NTIS database is a collection of more than 1.5 million titles, each of which is available for purchase. This database, which produces *Government Reports Announcements & Index* and *NTIS Alerts,* can be searched on CD-ROM and online through BRS, ORBIT, DIALOG, ESA-IRS, and STN.

6.3 *Government Reports Announcements & Index.* Springfield, VA, National Technical Information Service, April 4, 1975- . Biweekly with annual cumulations. Formerly: *Government Reports Announcements and Government Reports Index,* March 25, 1971-March 21,1975, biweekly; *U.S. Government Research and Development Reports,* January 5, 1965-March 10, 1971, biweekly; *U.S. Government Research and Development Reports Index,* 1968-March 10, 1971, biweekly, with quarterly and annual cumulations; *Government-wide Index to Federal Research & Development Reports,* monthly, 1965-66; biweekly, 1966-67.

6.4 *NTIS Alerts.* Springfield, VA, National Technical Information Service, 1973- . Twice a month. Formerly: *Abstract Newsletters; Weekly Government Abstracts.*

Government Reports Announcements & Index (GRA&I), published every two weeks by NTIS, includes complete bibliographic information and an abstract of the titles newly added to the database. The basic arrangement is by subject. Areas of particular interest to health sciences librarians are medicine and biology, behavior and society, agriculture and food, health care, biomedical technology and human factors engineering, and environmental pollution and control.

Each bibliographic entry identifies where the title may be obtained. Although copies of most reports are available from NTIS, some reports must be obtained from other agencies. The entry includes that information and, when available, specific instructions for ordering those reports.

NTIS Alerts are summaries of federally funded research in twenty-seven subject categories. The *Alerts* are published within a few weeks of NTIS receiving the reports from the originating agencies. With the exception of the first two topics, each subject area mentioned for *GRA&I* is an established category for *NTIS Alerts*. However, NTIS will customize an alert in any subject area, based on a user's specific needs.

National Aeronautics and Space Administration

The Scientific and Technical Information Facility of NASA maintains a database of more than 1.8 million references in the areas of aeronautics, space, and the supporting disciplines. Reports included in this database are abstracted in the NASA publication, *Scientific and Technical Aerospace Reports*.

> 6.5 *Scientific and Technical Aerospace Reports.* Washington, DC, National Aeronautics and Space Administration, 1963- . Biweekly; annual cumulative indexes.

Scientific and Technical Aerospace Reports (STAR) appears semimonthly and includes NASA, NASA contractor, and NASA grantee reports, plus other reports in the appropriate subject areas from both the governmental and private sectors. A companion journal, *International Aerospace Abstracts (IAA)*, announces journal, book, and conference literature.

STAR is available online through NASA/RECON. Its contents are also included in the Aerospace Database, which can be searched on CD-ROM and online through DIALOG.

Department of Energy

The Department of Energy (DOE) collects and disseminates information on nuclear science and technology. *Nuclear Science Abstracts*, which was published until June 30, 1976, included technical reports in its international coverage of the nuclear science literature.

> 6.6 *Energy Research Abstracts.* Oak Ridge, TN, U.S. Department of Energy, Office of Scientific and Technical Information, 1976- . Monthly, annual indexes.

Energy Research Abstracts (ERA), the successor to *Nuclear Science Abstracts*, provides coverage of materials relating to energy, including technical reports that were originated by DOE, any of its components, and its contractors. *ERA* appears monthly with annual indexes. Technical reports that have been included from DOE are available for purchase through NTIS. DOE's database—Energy, Science, and Technology—provides electronic access to *ERA*. The database is available online through DIALOG and STN, and also on CD-ROM.

Educational Resources Information Center

The Educational Resources Information Center (ERIC) is composed of a series of sixteen clearinghouses throughout the United States, each specializing in a different aspect of education. The clearinghouses are responsible for collecting and abstracting reports and other nonjournal literature. Acquisitions of the various clearinghouses are reported in *Resources in Education*.

6.7 Educational Resources Information Center. *Resources in Education.* Washington, DC, Office of Educational Research and Improvement, 1966- . Monthly. Formerly: *Research in Education.*

The monthly abstract journal includes reports and other nonjournal literature acquired by each of the sixteen clearinghouses. Documents cited in *Resources in Education* are available in paper copy and microfiche. The ERIC database can be searched on CD-ROM, and online service is provided through BRS and DIALOG.

British Library Document Supply Centre

One of the four divisions of the British Library, the Document Supply Centre is located at Boston Spa in Yorkshire. Among its extensive collections is a large report collection dating back to World War II. The BLDSC currently attempts to receive as many British reports as possible and has extensive holdings from other countries.

6.8 *British Reports, Translations, and Theses Received by the British Library Document Supply Centre.* Boston Spa, U.K., British Library Document Supply Centre, 1986- . Monthly. Formerly: *British Reports, Translations, and Theses,* 1981-1985; *BLLD Announcement Bulletin,* 1975-1980; *BLL Announcement Bulletin,* June 1973-December 1974; *NLL Announcement Bulletin,* 1971-May 1973; *British Research and Development Reports,* 1966-1971.

Since 1966, the British Library has listed reports from government and industry in the United Kingdom. Bibliographic information is provided in this monthly list, but no abstracts are available for the entries.

REFERENCES

1. Tallman J. History and importance of technical reports. Sci-Tech News 1961 Sum;15:46.
2. Information work with unpublished reports. Boulder, CO: Westview Press, 1977:61.

READINGS

U.S. Government Documents

Katz WA. Government documents. In: Introduction to reference work. Volume one: Basic information sources. 6th ed. New York: McGraw-Hill, 1992:425-54.

Morehead J, Fetzer M. Introduction to United States government information sources. 4th ed. Englewood, CO: Libraries Unlimited, 1992.

Taborsky T. CE 52: Government documents. Chicago: Medical Library Association, 1979.

Technical Reports

Grogan D. Research reports. In: Science and technology: An introduction to the literature. 4th ed. London: Clive Bingley, 1982:279-88.

Herner S, Herner M. The unpublished government research report: 1959 and 1985. Gov Pub R 1986 Jan-Feb;13:97-104.

Information work with unpublished reports. Boulder, CO: Westview Press, 1977:53-81.

McClure CR. The federal technical report literature: Research needs and issues. Gov Inf Q 1988;5(1):27-44.

Molholm KN et al. The defense technical information center: Acquiring information and imparting knowledge. Gov Inf Q 1988;5(4):323-40.

Morehead J, Fetzer M. Technical report literature and related research resources. In: Introduction to United States government information sources. 4th ed. Englewood, CO: Libraries Unlimited, 1992:351-404.

CHAPTER 7

Conferences, Reviews, and Translations

Fred W. Roper

CONFERENCES

Since World War II, meetings, conferences, and congresses have emerged as an increasingly important means of communication in the sciences. Similarly, the meeting has taken on a more important role in the social sciences as well. This situation has been equally true in the health sciences and in recent years the number of meetings has greatly increased.

These meetings are considered a major means for the exchange of information with colleagues and for the establishment of lines of professional communication. For the librarian, they pose several challenges. Patrons frequently want to know what, where, and when future meetings are planned. They might ask about the availability of papers that were presented or discussed at past meetings. Two major types of reference materials are needed to provide the information posed by these queries: calendars or lists of meetings to be held, and bibliographies of the published proceedings of meetings.

Calendars

Information on future meetings is available from a variety of sources. At a minimum, these sources should provide the sponsoring organization, name or topic of the meeting, the inclusive dates, the location, and, if possible, the name and address of a contact for additional information.

7.1 *Journal of the American Medical Association.* Chicago, American Medical Association, 1848- . Weekly.
7.2 *World Meetings: United States and Canada.* New York, Macmillan, 1963- . Quarterly.

7.3 *World Meetings: Outside United States and Canada.* New York, Macmillan, 1968- . Quarterly.

7.4 *World Meetings: Medicine.* New York, Macmillan, 1978- . Quarterly.

7.5 *Scientific Meetings.* San Diego, CA, Scientific Meetings Publications, 1957- . Quarterly.

7.6 *International Congress Calendar.* Brussels, Belgium, Union of International Associations, 1960- . Quarterly.

The *Journal of the American Medical Association (JAMA)* publishes reference directories in various issues on a variety of topics, including information on forthcoming meetings both inside and outside the United States. The Meetings in the United States directory appears in the first issue of each month; Meetings Outside the United States is published once in January and once in July. Meetings are announced up to one year in advance of the scheduled date. Each entry includes enough information so that the interested individual will be able to write for more complete program information. General medical periodicals and the journals of other organizations should also be consulted for calendars of meetings.

A number of publications give future meeting information for all the sciences. These publications are useful in health sciences libraries because physicians and researchers are likely to need information about meetings in other areas of the sciences.

Through two separate journals, World Meetings Publications "provide information on meetings of international, national, and regional interest in the sciences, applied sciences and engineering, social sciences, and professions" (Preface). *World Meetings: United States and Canada* and *World Meetings: Outside United States and Canada* represent the most comprehensive and detailed listings available of future meetings in the sciences. They are quarterly publications and contain information that is maintained in the World Meetings Data Base.

The main entry section is a two-year registry arranged into eight subsections, one for each quarter of the two-year period following the date of issue of the journal. In addition to the minimum expected information, a considerable amount of detail may be supplied, including restrictions on attendance, availability of papers, submission of papers deadlines, and a brief description of technical sessions. Entries are updated in succeeding issues as more information becomes available. Six indexes provide access to the main entries: keyword, location, date, publication, sponsor, and deadline for submission of abstracts or papers.

World Meetings: Medicine follows the same format and brings together in one publication all the entries relating to medicine and health found in the two general publications.

Scientific Meetings is a directory to future meetings of scientific, technical, and medical organizations. Coverage is international in scope, and it announces meetings scheduled in the coming fifteen months. The main section is a list of all meetings, arranged alphabetically by sponsoring agency. Each entry includes the inclusive dates, content of the meeting, and the name of a contact person. The subject index and chronological index provide access to the entries.

The Union of International Associations provides coverage of international meetings in all disciplines through its *International Congress Calendar.* The *Calendar* contains information for meetings that will take place in the coming twelve to fifteen months, and for meetings planned up to ten years in advance. The descriptions are listed in a geographical section by country and city, and in a chronological section. A single index based on keywords in the organization name, conference name, or the conference theme refers to both sections.

Although the primary purpose of these tools is to identify future meetings, they are often used to establish that a meeting was scheduled to take place. In addition to these current tools, there are retrospective lists of the meetings that have been held. These lists may include information about publications resulting from the meetings.

7.7 *Congresses: Tentative Chronological and Bibliographical Reference List of National and International Meetings of Physicians, Scientists and Experts.* Washington, DC, U.S. Government Printing Office, 1938. Supplement to *Index Catalogue,* 4th series, 2d supplement.

7.8 Council for International Organizations of Medical Sciences. *Bibliography of International Congresses of Medical Sciences.* Springfield, IL, Charles C. Thomas, Publisher, 1958.

7.9 *International Congresses, 1681 to 1899, Full List.* Brussels, Belgium, Union of International Associations, 1960. Documents, no. 8: Publication no. 164.

7.10 *International Congresses, 1900 to 1919, Full List.* Brussels, Belgium, Union of International Associations, 1964. Publication no. 188.

A supplement to the *Index Catalogue* in 1938, *Congresses: Tentative Chronological and Bibliographical Reference List of National and International Meetings of Physicians, Scientists and Experts* provides information on 17,000 congresses that was available in the Army Medical Library. For some of the congresses very little is available beyond the fact that the congress was held and the date. For others there may be a detailed listing of the individual sessions and information about any resulting publications.

The list from the *Index Catalogue* includes those congresses that are of peripheral interest to researchers in the health sciences as well as those that are in direct relationship. In 1958, the *Bibliography of International Congresses of Medical Sciences* was published under the auspices of the Council for International Organizations of Medical Sciences. This list includes only those congresses directly related to the medical sciences; 1,427 congresses in the field of medicine are identified. The basic arrangement is a chronological listing by subject.

The Union of International Associations has prepared two lists of international congresses covering all subject areas from 1681 to 1899 and from 1900 to 1919. Each provides a chronological approach, giving the name of the congress, its location, and the date. *International Congresses, 1900 to 1919, Full List* includes a subject index for both volumes.

Papers Presented at Meetings

The papers presented or discussed at meetings often represent the latest and most up-to-date information available on a topic. For the librarian, there is the difficulty of identifying the presenter, the title of the paper, and whether or not the paper has been published.

Cruzat [1] has identified six major forms of presentation for the proceedings of meetings.

1. A multivolume work encompassing the total proceedings of a conference or meeting.
2. A monograph or report with a specific title and editor.
3. A supplement, special number, or entire issue of an established journal because it is one of the official publications of the society or agency that organized the meeting, or because of the subject content of an individual symposium or conference the society or agency elects to publish it.
4. Selected papers or abstracts published in a journal because it is the official organ or because of subject content.
5. Reports of a meeting or conference in a journal that has a special section devoted to "congress or conference proceedings."
6. Dual publication as both an issue or part of a journal and as a monograph or report.

In addition, the individual papers may be submitted to appropriate journals for separate publication. These papers will then be included in the indexing and abstracting services that index the journals.

A problem of identification arises when the paper has been revised and published under another title. Identification is further complicated by the current practice of taping proceedings. These tapes, which may be the only record of a meeting, are not likely to be included in the traditional bibliographic sources.

7.11 *Conference Papers Index*. Bethesda, MD, Cambridge Scientific Abstracts, 1973- . Monthly. Formerly: *Current Programs*.

Published since 1973, *Conference Papers Index (CPI)* provides a listing of all the papers presented at meetings, whether or not the paper appeared in published format. This source covers scientific meetings, including those in the health sciences, and is prepared mainly from programs or abstract publications of the conferences. *CPI* is arranged by topic into seventeen sections. Six of these sections—including pharmacology, clinical medicine, and experimental medicine—are of direct interest to researchers in the life sciences. Information on publications resulting from the meeting is indicated, as is the name and address of the individual presenters. This source is particularly useful when a preprint distributed either before or at the meeting is the only known publication of a particular paper. *Conference Papers Index* can be searched online through DIALOG, ESA-IRS, and STN.

Current Bibliographies of Published Proceedings

The published proceedings may include either full text or just an abstract of the papers presented at meetings. Some proceedings will include everything presented at the meeting and others will be selective. There are several bibliographic sources, most of them covering all the sciences, that list published proceedings on a regular basis.

7.12 *Index to Scientific and Technical Proceedings*. Philadelphia, Institute for Scientific Information, 1978- . Monthly, annual cumulation.

7.13 *Directory of Published Proceedings: Series SEMT—Science/ Engineering/Medicine/Technology*. Harrison, NY, InterDok, 1965- . Ten issues per year, annual cumulation. *Cumulated Index Supplement*. Harrison, NY, InterDok. Quarterly, annual cumulation.

7.14 *Directory of Published Proceedings: Series PCE—Pollution Control/Ecology*. Harrison, NY, InterDok, 1974- . Annual.

7.15 *Proceedings in Print*. Halifax, MA, Proceedings in Print, Inc., 1964- . Six issues per year; annual cumulative index.

Index to Scientific and Technical Proceedings (ISTP) covers published proceedings in all the sciences. It is produced by the Institute for Scientific Information (ISI) and includes materials selected from ISI's various databases. Approximately 30% of the materials are in the life sciences. The proceedings, regardless of the format in which they appeared, must contain complete papers to be listed in *ISTP;* proceedings that include both complete papers and abstracts are also included. Many indexing services index only proceedings volumes, but *ISTP* indexes the individual papers. Published monthly, *ISTP* offers one of the fastest means of access to the proceedings literature.

The main section of *ISTP* provides complete bibliographic information for the published proceedings. The entry includes titles of papers, authors, and address of the first author in cases of multiple authorship. The category index and the permuterm subject index provide a subject approach. The sponsors of the meetings are found in the sponsor index. The author/editor index and the corporate index give access to the authors of papers, editors of the proceedings, and corporate affiliations of individual authors. The meetings location index provides country and city where the meeting was held. *ISTP* is also available online through DIMDI.

InterDok Corporation is responsible for two bibliographies of scientific meetings—*Directory of Published Proceedings: Series SEMT* and *Directory of Published Proceedings: Series PCE.* They provide basic bibliographic information for proceedings that have been identified in their respective areas of responsibility. Since 1964, *Series SEMT* has provided monthly information on preprints and published proceedings of international congresses, conferences, symposia, meetings, seminars, and summer schools. Its principal arrangement for entries is chronological by date of meeting, with indexes by subject/sponsor, location, and editor. *Series PCE,* issued annually, is prepared from the entries in *Series SEMT* and a companion publication, *Series SSH—Social Sciences/Humanities.*

Proceedings in Print is broader in scope than the above titles; it covers all subject areas. Conferences can be identified through the alphabetical index, which uses headings found in the proceedings: corporate author, sponsoring agency, editor, and subject.

Because of the information provided, these current bibliographies of proceedings serve both as a means of verifying that a particular conference took place and as acquisitions sources. Once a meeting's publications have been identified, it is then possible to acquire the proceedings, by using either the information provided in the bibliographies or other sources to locate a library that may hold them.

7.16 *Index of Conference Proceedings.* Boston Spa, U.K., British Library Document Supply Centre. No. 69- , June 1973- . Monthly. *Index of Conference Proceedings. Annual Cumulation.* 1988- . Continues: *Index of Conference Proceedings Received. Annual Cumulation.* 1985-1987.

7.17 *Index of Conference Proceedings 1964-1988.* London, Saur, 1989.

One of the most comprehensive collections of proceedings in the world is located at the British Library Document Supply Centre. More than 300,000 citations to proceedings of conferences, congresses, symposia, workshops, and seminars are in the collection. *Index of Conference Proceedings* includes proceedings published in monographs or parts of reports, and in journals. The monthly publication is arranged alphabetically by subject keywords taken from the titles and organizers of the proceedings. Under each of the keywords there is a chronological listing of all the appropriate conferences and the published proceedings. The collection includes all subject areas, but emphasis is on the sciences. The *Index* is available online through BLAISE-LINE and on CD-ROM.

The *Index of Conference Proceedings 1964-1988* is a cumulation of the proceedings acquired during the 25-year period.

In addition to these titles that are specifically concerned with proceedings of meetings, the librarian must consult indexing and abstracting services for periodical coverage of proceedings and individual papers given at meetings. Sources for monographs, such as the *National Library of Medicine Current Catalog* and the *National Union Catalog*, will provide coverage of separately published proceedings.

REVIEWS

In an era of interdisciplinary research that requires the synthesis of information from a variety of sources, reviews of research in the health sciences are vital forms of scientific communication. The review brings together information about previously published research and provides the researcher with an overview of work that has been carried out in a particular area. Through reviews, the primary literature may be reduced to a more manageable state.

For the student, the review may serve as an introduction to a topic; for the practicing scientist, it may function as a guide to a field that is only of peripheral interest. The researcher in the field will find the review useful to identify items that may have been previously overlooked or to update knowledge.

A review usually cites a large number of references and is confined to examining the literature already published rather than presenting new information. Often the title will include an identifier such as "review of," "progress in," "advances in," or "yearbook of."

Typically, reviews are found in two formats. One is the serial publication devoted to review-type articles, e.g., *Annual Review of Medicine, Biological Reviews, Progress in Clinical Pathology*, and *Year Book of Surgery*. The other is in the form of individual articles found in the primary sources of information, such as books, periodicals, and technical report literature. A review may also appear in the form of a literature search that is performed by a scientist in preparation of a research study. However, it is usually more difficult to gain access to this type of review.

Bibliographic control of reviews in the health sciences has generally surpassed that in the other sciences, due in large part to the efforts of the National Library of Medicine. Other agencies have routinely included and identified review publications in indexing and abstracting activities as well.

> 7.18 *Bibliography of Medical Reviews.* Bethesda, MD, National Library of Medicine, 1955- . Annual, 1955-1967. Monthly, 1968-1977, separately and in *Index Medicus.* Monthly, 1978- , only in *Index Medicus.*
>
> 7.19 *Index to Scientific Reviews.* Philadelphia, PA, Institute for Scientific Information, 1974- . Semiannual.

The primary purpose of these two publications is to identify reviews. The first source deals with the health sciences and the second includes all branches of science.

The *Bibliography of Medical Reviews (BMR)* is a continuing feature of *Index Medicus (IM).* BMR first appeared in 1955 as an annual publication; a six-year cumulation in 1961 represents review articles from the *1955-59 Current List of Medical Literature* and the *1960 Cumulated Index Medicus (CIM).* It continued as an annual publication through 1967; since January 1968, it has been published as a part of the monthly *IM* with an annual cumulation in *CIM.* It was also published as a separate monthly publication from 1968 through 1977. Since January 1978, *BMR* has appeared only as a separate section of *Index Medicus.*

Bibliography of Medical Reviews follows the same format as *IM* and provides subject access to citations to reviews. In 1988, NLM expanded its definition of medical reviews to include categories of materials that were previously excluded from *BMR.* The definition now includes articles such as academic reviews, subject reviews, epidemiologic reviews, and state-of-the-art reviews. Online access to *BMR* is provided through MEDLINE.

Since 1974, the Institute for Scientific Information (ISI) has published the *Index to Scientific Reviews (ISR)* to provide separate bibliographic coverage of the world's scientific review literature. *ISR* is a semiannual publication that draws from the databases used to produce other ISI publications. It represents the most comprehensive coverage of the review literature for all of the sciences. In addition to monographic review series and review journals, *ISR* includes review articles retrieved from SCISEARCH, the *Science Citation Index (SCI)* database.

ISR serves both as a source of bibliographic information for the reviews currently being published and as a citation index to these articles. The main section of *ISR* is the research front specialty index, which provides bibliographies of current reviews in identified areas of intense research activity. This section is accessed using the source index and permuterm subject index. The corporate index is arranged by authors' geographic location and organizational affiliations. *ISR* can be searched on the *SCI* and *SciSearch* CD-ROMs and online as a part of the SCISEARCH database through DIALOG, DIMDI, and Data-Star.

> 7.20 *Biological Abstracts/RRM (Reports/Reviews/Meetings)*. Philadelphia, PA, BioSciences Information Service, 1980- . Monthly; semiannual index.

In 1980, *Biological Abstracts/RRM (BA/RRM)* succeeded the BioSciences Information Service (BIOSIS) publication, *BioResearch Index*. BA/RRM covers the nontraditional forms of literature in the life sciences with particular attention to reports, reviews, and meetings. The monthly publication contains citations to a wide variety of formats that are not normally found in indexing and abstracting services or that have had limited coverage in the past. *BA/RRM* can be searched on CD-ROM and online through BRS, DIALOG, Data-Star, STN, and ESA-IRS as part of the BIOSIS Previews database.

In addition to these three sources, which are designed specifically for the bibliographic control of reviews, other tools should be consulted. Citations to reviews are included in various indexing and abstracting services, some of which provide an indicator that the item cited is a review.

TRANSLATIONS

The promotion and stimulation of scientific progress and development depend on effective communication among the world's scientists. Frequently this communication is hindered by the language barrier. Significant research results published in a language unfamiliar to a scientist have limited value. This situation exists with the biomedical literature as well as with that of other subject areas.

There are several options available when a research article has been published in a foreign language. On an informal level, the researcher may have someone either partially or completely translate the article to determine if a formal translation is worthwhile. On a more formal level there are three primary methods available: translation clearinghouses, cover-to-cover translations, and translation agencies or freelance translators.

Dealing with the bibliographic control of translations is a relatively recent development. No centralized translation service existed in the United States prior to World War II. Consequently, it was necessary for the scientist to either read foreign-language articles in the original language or to personally secure translations. With more global awareness in the scientific community, there is the conviction that access to foreign scientific writing is a necessity. This conviction has been heightened since World War II and particularly since the launching of Sputnik by the USSR in 1957. Today more than 50% of the world's scientific and technical information is published in languages other than English [2]. Particular interest has developed in publications from Eastern Europe, Russia, Japan, and the People's Republic of China.

It is unlikely that scientists will develop greater fluency in foreign languages; as a result, their dependence on translations is likely to continue and even to increase. Cost is an important factor in the production of translations, and there have been attempts to share this expense in various ways, usually through publication of the translations or providing bibliographic access to a collection of translations.

Translation Centers

Translation centers serve as a central collecting point for translations that have been made for individuals and organizations. Translations are deposited with the center, which then provides bibliographic access to the information and may also offer reference service.

United States: The National Translations Center (NTC) was the primary national resource for English-language translations in the natural, physical, medical, and social sciences. Last located at the Library of Congress, the program was unable to attain cost recovery; consequently, the decision was made to discontinue the service and the NTC closed on September 30, 1993 [3].

NTC began after World War II as an effort of the Science-Technology Division of the Special Libraries Association (SLA). Members of the division collected unpublished translations and maintained a union catalog. In 1953, NTC was formally organized at the John Crerar Library. It continued its association with the SLA until it became an independent department of the John Crerar Library in 1970. As a part of a merger in 1984, NTC moved to the University of Chicago. In 1989, the center's materials were transferred to the Library of Congress, where it was a unit of the Cataloging Distribution Service.

Information on the location of nearly 1 million translations—approximately 400,00 are held at LC—is contained in the NTC files. This collection comprises translations of journal articles, patents, conference papers, and other forms of technical literature. Translations were received from scientific and professional societies, government agencies, special libraries, corporations, universities, and other institutions.

NTC acquired and cataloged machine-readable records for more than 31,000 translations when it was a part of the Library of Congress. Those records can be searched through bibliographic utilities such as OCLC and WLN. However, at the time of publication of this book, it was unknown if LC would be able to sustain availability of the translations cited in those databases.

7.21 *Translations Register-Index.* Chicago, National Translations Center, John Crerar Library, 1967-1986. Continued by: *World Translations Index,* 1987-1988.

7.22 National Translations Center. *Consolidated Index of Translations into English.* New York, Special Libraries Association, 1969.

7.23 *Consolidated Index of Translations into English II: 1967-1984.* Chicago, National Translations Center, 1986. 3 vols.

The *Translations Register-Index* is the bibliographic source for translations acquired by NTC from 1967 through 1986. The register section lists translations according to subject categories. The index section comprises journal citations and patent citations. Journals are listed alphabetically by title, followed by the year, volume, issue, and pages that are available in translation. Patents are arranged by country, and the directory is used to determine from which source the patent is available. The cumulated index includes NTC acquisitions that have been announced in the register section. NTC ceased publication of the *Translations Register-Index* and joined with the International Translation Centre for 1987 and 1988 to publish its holdings in *World Translations Index* (*see* 7.26).

For information on translations made available from 1953 through 1966, the *Consolidated Index of Translations into English* (*CITE I*) should be consulted. More than 142,000 translations are included. This publication is a cumulation of previously published lists from the Library of Congress, the Special Libraries Association, NTC, and a number of specialized sources.

The *Consolidated Index of Translations into English II* (*CITE II*) cumulates citation information on an additional 250,00 translations of scientific and technical journals previously listed in *Translations Register-Index.*

The translations announced in these three indexes are located at the Library of Congress.

United Kingdom: The British Library Document Supply Centre (BLDSC) is the largest depository of translations in the United Kingdom and one of the largest in the world. In addition to collecting translations, BLDSC has actively promoted cover-to-cover translations of Russian-language periodicals.

7.24 *British Reports, Translations, and Theses Received by the British Library Document Supply Centre.* Boston Spa, U.K., British Library Document Supply Centre, 1986- . Monthly. Formerly: *British Reports, Translations, and Theses*, 1981-1985; *BLLD Announcement Bulletin*, 1975-1980; *BLL Announcement Bulletin*, June 1973-December 1974; *NLL Announcement Bulletin*, 1971-May 1973; *British Research and Development Reports*, 1966-1971.

British Reports, Translations, and Theses is a monthly listing of both technical report literature and translations acquired by the British Library. All items are held at BLDSC and photocopies may be obtained if copyright allows, or the item will be loaned out.

International: The International Translations Centre, located at Delft in The Netherlands, functioned from 1961 until 1976 as the European Translations Centre. The name was changed to better reflect the scope of the organization. Both the U.S. and the United Kingdom centers concentrate on translations from a foreign language into English; the International Translations Centre collects translations into all languages.

7.25 *World Transindex.* Delft, The Netherlands, International Translations Centre, 1978-1986.

7.26 *World Translations Index.* Delft, The Netherlands, International Translations Centre, 1987- . 10 issues per year. Continues: *Translations Register-Index*, 1987-1988; and *World Transindex.*

In 1978, *World Transindex* succeeded *World Index of Scientific Translations and List of Translations Notified to the International Translation Centre, Transatom Bulletin,* and *Bulletin des Traductions.* It is a subject listing with author and source indexes; all subject areas and languages are represented.

World Translations Index "announces translations of literature relating to all fields of science and technology, from all languages into Western languages" (Introduction). The reference section lists bibliographic details of the translation and of the original article, location where the translation may be obtained, journals containing the translation, or translations commercially issued as monographs. This section is accessed by an author index and a subject index, which cites bibliographic information of the original publications. The indexes are cumulated annually and published in a separate volume. *World Translations Index* is available online through DIALOG.

Cover-to-Cover Translations

These publications, usually serial in nature, may enter into the normal channels of bibliography and may be indexed as a matter of course in the major indexing and abstracting services. For the librarian, it may be difficult to determine the availability of a journal that is translated on a regular basis. *Ulrich's International Periodicals Directory, New Serial Titles, Chemical Abstracts Service Source Index,* and *World Translations Index* will be useful tools in identifying the journals that are regularly translated. Once this is determined, the next step is to find out which indexing and abstracting services include the translated journal.

7.27 Himmelsbach, Carl J., and Brociner, Grace E. *A Guide to Scientific and Technical Journals in Translation.* 2d ed. New York, Special Libraries Association, 1972.

A Guide to Scientific and Technical Journals in Translation provides a listing of those journals that are completely or partially translated and indicates the source for obtaining them. There is also a guide to the volumes that have appeared in translation.

7.28 *Journals in Translation.* 5th ed. Boston Spa, U.K., British Library Document Supply Centre; Delft, The Netherlands, International Translations Centre, 1991.

The International Translations Centre and the British Library Document Supply Centre jointly publish *Journals in Translation,* which is a bibliography of periodicals that are completely or partially translated. Most of the translations are into English. The scope of this publication includes all subject areas, but emphasis is on the sciences.

Cover-to-cover translations of journals originally published in a foreign language represent a significant portion of the translation industry. Bishop and Pukteris [4] give a detailed description of such translations with regard to the literature of the health sciences. They note the expense involved in the production and acquisition of the cover-to-cover translations.

REFERENCES

1. Cruzat GS. Keeping up with biomedical meetings. RQ 1967 Fall;7:12-20.
2. National translations center is now OCLC document supplier. ALCTS News 1992 3(7):86.
3. Librarian makes organizational, personnel changes. LC Inf Bull 1993 Sept;52(16):322.

4. Bishop D, Pukteris S. English translations of biomedical journal literature: availability and control. Bull Med Libr Assoc 1973 Jan;61:24-28.

READINGS

Conferences

Cruzat GS. Keeping up with biomedical meetings. RQ 1967 Fall;7:12-20.

Grogan D. Conference proceedings. In: Science and technology: an introduction to the literature. 4th ed. London: Clive Bingley, 1982:262-78.

Mills PR. Characteristics of published conference proceedings. Jour Doc 1973 Mar;29:36-50.

Reviews

Grogan D. Reviews of progress. In: Science and technology: an introduction to the literature. 4th ed. London: Clive Bingley, 1982:249-61.

Manten AA. Scientific review literature. Schol pub 1973 Oct;5:75-89.

Virgo JA. The review article: its characteristics and problems. Lib Q 1971 Oct;41:275-91.

Translations

Bishop D, Pukteris S. English translations of biomedical journal literature: availability and control. Bull Med Libr Assoc 1973 Jan;61:24-28.

Chan FKL. The foreign language barrier in science and technology. Int Lib Rev 1976 June;8:317-25.

Chillage JP. Translations and their guides. NLL Rev 1971 Apr;1:46-53.

Fedunok S. Printed and online sources for technical translations. Science and technology libraries 1982 Winter;3:3-12.

Grogan D. Translations. In: Science and technology: an introduction to the literature. 4th ed. London: Clive Bingley, 1982:324-37.

PART III

Information Sources

CHAPTER 8

Terminology

Taylor Putney and Fred W. Roper

To understand the literature of the health sciences, it is important to know the specialized terminology that characterizes it. This vocabulary is accessed through a variety of reference works, each one designed to answer a particular type of question, teach a particular part of the vocabulary, or provide a specific piece of information. Terminology reference tools may be grouped by type: comprehensive dictionaries of the health sciences; specialized dictionaries, such as those for abbreviations or etymology; terminology textbooks; specialized subject dictionaries; foreign-language dictionaries; and compilations of syndromes and eponyms.

GENERAL DICTIONARIES

An unabridged medical dictionary is first and foremost a record of the use of medical terminology. In a world where new diseases, new operations, new procedures, and new syndromes are continuously being discovered and named, dictionaries must be updated regularly. A dictionary should reflect the terminology that is currently in use in the medical professions. To serve this need, there are two unabridged medical dictionaries that are extensively used in the United States.

8.1 *Dorland's Illustrated Medical Dictionary.* 27th ed. Philadelphia, PA, Saunders, 1988.
8.2 *Stedman's Medical Dictionary.* 25th ed. Baltimore, MD, Williams & Wilkins, 1990.

Now in its 27th edition, *Dorland's Illustrated Medical Dictionary* is considered by many to be the "dean of medical dictionaries." It is comprehensive, authoritative, and has been a standby for many years. *Dorland's* contains more than 1,850 pages of definitions and many special features, foremost of which is the "Fundamentals of Medical Etymology" section. This brief introduction to the formation of medical terms includes lists of the most used prefixes, suffixes, and root words. In addition to the usual dictionary illustrations, there are twenty-nine tables and fifty-three plates, all of which appear in alphabetical order.

In an effort to avoid printing the same definition many times, the editors of *Dorland's* have made extensive use of cross-references for words that are synonyms. The preferred term is defined and synonyms are referenced to that term. Also, anatomical terms are defined only under their official names, with cross-references from common names. A major feature of word arrangement is the use of subentries. Definitions of the variations of the main entry are found in the same paragraph as a main entry. Each subentry appears in boldface type in the body of the paragraph headed by the main entry. The dictionary uses letter-by-letter alphabetization of words and abbreviations.

Stedman's Medical Dictionary is similar to *Dorland's* and is accepted by many as equal in authority and content. The 25th edition has been completely revised by thirty-six consultants and five contributors. A useful feature of *Stedman's* is the opening section describing how to use the dictionary, including guides to pronunciation, derivations, abbreviations, and spelling of medical terms.

The alphabetizing of terms and the main entry/subentry arrangement are very similar to *Dorland's*. The subentry locator, which precedes section A of the vocabulary, lists all of the subentries used in the text of the dictionary. The subentry is followed by the main entries under which it can be found. *Stedman's* also makes frequent use of cross-references to avoid duplicating definitions. Furthermore, there are many "see" references that direct the reader to related information. Eponyms and anatomical, chemical, biochemical, and pharmacological terms are included as main entries.

Stedman's is well illustrated, including 126 tables placed throughout the textbook and twenty-four color plates grouped in the center. It also includes a guide to medical etymology that contains lists of roots. The contrasting typefaces make it easy to locate and read entries.

A great deal of information not usually found in a dictionary is provided in the five appendices: a summary of blood groups, temperature equivalents, comparative temperature scales, weights and measures, and laboratory reference values. The complete text of *Stedman's* is also available electronically as Stedman's/25 for WordPerfect.

Dorland's and *Stedman's* are very similar in size, authority, and comprehensiveness. Each is revised on a regular basis. Today's computer technology allows for faster updating of dictionaries and reduced time between revision and publication.

However, even with regular revisions, no editorial board will arrive at a completely comprehensive list of medical terms. Determining which terms to delete because they are obsolete, imprecise, or no longer commonly used, and which new terms to include because they are now widely used, is a subjective editorial decision. Consequently, each dictionary contains definitions that the other excludes. All but perhaps the very smallest libraries should have both of these dictionaries in their collections to ensure the broadest coverage of vocabulary and special features.

> 8.3 *Blakiston's Gould Medical Dictionary.* 4th ed. New York, McGraw-Hill, 1979.

Blakiston's Gould Medical Dictionary has not been updated since the fourth edition was published in 1979. Although not as well known as either *Dorland's* or *Stedman's*, it is nevertheless an important unabridged dictionary. The major difference between it and the previously discussed dictionaries is in terms of format. *Blakiston's* contains no subentries, but rather alphabetizes all terms and their subparts letter-by-letter. Synonyms are defined by the preferred term, and the preferred term is defined in full. There are no entry illustrations, but there are plates grouped together in the middle of the textbook. Like the other unabridged dictionaries, *Blakiston's* includes a brief guide to medical etymology. Also, like *Stedman's*, *Blakiston's* includes a number of very useful appendices.

> 8.4 *Butterworths Medical Dictionary.* 2d ed. London, Butterworths, 1978.

A comparable title to the preceding three is the second edition of *Butterworths Medical Dictionary.* It is similar to the three American dictionaries in vocabulary and comprehensiveness, but emphasis is on British use.

Just as there are unabridged and abridged English-language dictionaries, there are both types of medical dictionaries. There are four abridged medical dictionaries of particular importance.

> 8.5 *Taber's Cyclopedic Medical Dictionary.* 17th ed. Philadelphia, PA, Davis, 1993.
> 8.6 *Black's Medical Dictionary.* 37th ed. Lanham, MD, Barnes and Noble, 1992.
> 8.7 *The Bantam Medical Dictionary.* New York, Bantam Books, 1990. Previously published as: *Urdang Dictionary of Current Medical Terms.*
> 8.8 Dox, Ida; Melloni, B. John; and Eisner, Gilbert. *The HarperCollins Illustrated Medical Dictionary.* New York, HarperPerennial, 1993. New

edition of: *Melloni's Illustrated Medical Dictionary.* 2d ed. Baltimore, MD, Williams & Wilkins, 1985.

Taber's Cyclopedic Medical Dictionary states that it is "an abridged dictionary intended for all persons in nursing and allied health fields" (Introduction). It includes all the standard features of an unabridged dictionary but defines fewer words. However, it provides much information not found in an unabridged dictionary, and most definitions are encyclopedic in scope. For example, the entry "cerebrospinal fluid" includes paragraphs on the formation and characteristics of the fluid.

A unique feature of *Taber's* is the "interpreter," which is a list of questions and statements that might be used in patient examination translated into five languages. In addition, there is a fact-finding index that lists terms that have the following subheadings: diagnosis, etiology, first-aid, nursing implications, poisoning, prognosis, treatment, caution, and signs/symptoms. There are 357 pages of appendices that include tables, charts, and supplementary information on units of measurement, abbreviations, nomenclature, anatomy, drug interactions, and medical emergencies. *Taber's* also provides directories of burn centers and poison control centers.

Taber's is a good dictionary for paramedical personnel and others who need a medical dictionary but do not need the complexity and expense of one of the unabridged dictionaries.

The purpose of *Black's Medical Dictionary* "...is to provide a concise and understandable text in medicine's many aspects" (Preface). *Black's* is written for the nonprofessional who must have some basic knowledge of medicine to interact intelligently with the physician. It contains main entries in boldface type, usually followed by long articles on the subject. Broad topics, such as "Insects in relation to disease," "Injured, removal of," and "Drowning, recovery from," are discussed at length.

Although "see" references are used to link various topics, there is still considerable duplication of definitions. For example, there is a discussion of the thyroid gland under "endocrine glands" as well as under the main entry. *Black's* is distinctly different from the other dictionaries discussed because the format and style are designed to be easily accessible to the layperson.

The Bantam Medical Dictionary and *The HarperCollins Illustrated Medical Dictionary* are two examples of a growing number of general dictionaries that include unique special features.

The Bantam Medical Dictionary provides full definitions for terms in the basic sciences as well as the major specialties such as community medicine, psychology, and surgery. Special features within the definitions include subentries; "see" cross-references; and starred words, which are entered and defined in their own alphabetical places. The dictionary contains about 150 fully labeled illustrations.

The HarperCollins is written for the general public and students in the health sciences. It includes brief definitions of more than 26,000 terms and uses 2,500 illustrations to supplement the text. The illustrations and terms illustrated appear on the same page. It is the most heavily illustrated dictionary available.

MEDICAL ETYMOLOGY

Etymology is important to anyone using medical terminology because it explains how words were formed. Today's medical vocabulary is based on Greek and Latin prefixes, roots, and suffixes; therefore, the definition of a medical word is a combination of the definitions of its prefix, root or roots, and suffix. If one knows the definitions of these parts, one can define the word. The importance of understanding a word's parts is demonstrated by the fact that a section on medical etymology is included in each of the major medical dictionaries discussed earlier.

8.9 Skinner, Henry Alan. *Origin of Medical Terms*. Reprint. New York, Hafner, 1970.

8.10 Haubrich, William S. *Medical Meanings: A Glossary of Word Origins*. 1st ed. San Diego, Harcourt Brace Jovanovich, 1984.

8.11 Jaeger, Edmund C. *A Source-Book of Biological Names and Terms*. 3d ed. Springfield, IL, Thomas, 1955.

Origin of Medical Terms is a general reference work of medical terms directed primarily at the beginning medical student. It is strongest in the basic sciences vocabulary. The book has a readable format and provides references to books or articles introducing new terms. Skinner explains some eponyms but discourages their use. One slight drawback for Americans is that the book generally uses British spellings.

Skinner's work is no longer in print, but *Medical Meanings: A Glossary of Word Origins* is intended to fill this gap in medical source material. The meanings of terms have been updated, new terms are described, and origins other than those more commonly associated with the terms are explored. *Medical Meanings* is an alphabetical list of principal words and important prefixes and suffixes. The index contains terms that are subentries; principal words that appear in more than one entry; and categories of words (e.g., colors, phobias) that are grouped together.

Jaeger's *Source-Book* is more complex than the works by Skinner and Haubrich and covers a wider range of words; hence the word "biological" rather than "medical" in the title. The third edition includes a textbook and a supplement that is fully cross-referenced to the main volume. The textbook's opening section includes information about how words are formed, types of words, and an abbreviation guide. Both volumes are arranged alphabetically. Each entry defines the word parts and makes reference to the supplement if necessary. Numerous examples are given and some geographical and personal names are included.

TERMINOLOGY TEXTBOOKS

There are many textbooks that teach the student or health professional the basics of medical terminology. These books employ various methods and are arranged in various formats. However, most current terminology textbooks have the same goal: To teach the student the basic word parts (prefixes, roots, combining forms, and suffixes) that form medical terms.

This section describes two textbooks that differ in their approach, in order to show the range of choices available to the individual who wants to learn medical vocabulary.

> 8.12 Austrin, Miriam G. and Austrin, Harvey R. *Learning Medical Terminology.* 7th ed. Revised edition of *Young's Learning Medical Terminology.* St. Louis, MO, Mosby, 1991.
>
> 8.13 Smith, Genevieve L. and David, Phyllis E. *Medical Terminology: A Programmed Text.* 6th ed. Revised by Jean T. Dennerll. Albany, NY, Delmar, 1991.

Learning Medical Terminology is designed for students to use as a combination textbook and workbook. It begins with the components needed to build a medical vocabulary and includes tables of prefixes, suffixes, combining forms, verbal and adjectival derivatives, body fluids, body systems, and colors. Following these introductory chapters are individual chapters on each body system. A chapter typically begins with a textual description of the body system; terms are introduced; and the written description is supplemented with diagrams and illustrations. A glossary of terms and a set of exercises on the material presented follows the textual description. There are a number of appendices, including abbreviations and symbols, medical specialties, and hospital reports.

In contrast, *Medical Terminology: A Programmed Text* is designed to teach medical terminology through repetitive use of prefixes, suffixes, and combining forms. In more than 1,650 frames, the student repeatedly answers questions and fills in blank spaces with the proper prefix, root, combining form, suffix, or definition. The student who knows word parts will be able to use that knowledge to define unfamiliar terms. The book is intended for individuals working in medical fields and for those whose work brings them in contact with medical terms on a regular basis. It has been used successfully in classes for allied health professionals and medical secretaries also.

Medical Terminology can be adapted for classroom use because the frames are conveniently divided into sections appropriate for individual assignments. In addition, there are fifty-six review activity sheets for student use. Special features include a glossary of word parts used in the text, with references to the frame in which each first appears. Also included are many anatomical illustrations and a list of medical abbreviations.

A unique feature of *Medical Terminology* is the series of audiotapes, available separately from the publisher, that accompany the textbook. The tapes provide another method to study the word parts and allow the student to hear the proper pronunciation of each word part.

MEDICAL ABBREVIATIONS

The use of abbreviations and acronyms has proliferated in the health sciences, and one recurrent problem is that a single abbreviation may have a number of different meanings. For example, PPV may stand for "positive-pressure ventilation" or "progressive pneumonia virus." Conversely, multiple abbreviations may exist for a single term. It is essential for the reference collection to have up-to-date sources that list the possible meanings of acronyms and abbreviations.

8.14 Jablonski, Stanley. *Dictionary of Medical Acronyms and Abbreviations.* 2d ed. Philadelphia, PA, Hanley & Belfus, 1993.

8.15 *Stedman's Abbreviations, Acronyms, and Symbols.* Baltimore, MD, Williams & Wilkins, 1992.

8.16 Mitchell-Hatton, Sarah Lu. *The Davis Book of Medical Abbreviations: A Deciphering Guide.* Philadelphia, PA, Davis, 1991.

8.17 Kerr, Avice H. *Medical Hieroglyphs.* Downey, CA, Enterprise Publications, 1970.

Jablonski's *Dictionary* lists the most frequently used acronyms and abbreviations that were identified by screening NLM's collection of books and periodicals. No definitions are given, only the full entry of possible meanings for the terms.

The *Stedman's* compilation was produced by reviewing dictionaries, "approved lists" from teaching hospitals, and other compendia. Although more than 20,000 clinically relevant terms are listed, there is less overlapping than might be expected between this source and Jablonski's. A comparison of the terms listed between LD and LH indicates considerable differences in the number of terms and the number of possible meanings.

The Davis Book of Medical Abbreviations: A Deciphering Guide is a useful tool because it contains obsolete, profane, slang, and nonmedical abbreviations. It includes pronunciations of acronyms and words that have been crafted from abbreviations (e.g., "trick" for Trichomonas), enabling the user to identify an unknown term. It deciphers medical codes by the use of medical specialty listings that appear after the full entry (e.g., Trichomonas [lab]).

Medical Hieroglyphs contains abbreviations taken directly from medical records. Hence, it contains abbreviations that are standard or universally accepted. This book also includes a section on symbols used by physicians.

WORD FINDERS AND CONCEPT DICTIONARIES

Most dictionaries consist of alphabetical lists of words followed by definitions. This arrangement is adequate if one knows the word. However, when only a definition or concept is known, a dictionary that uses words as the access point is useless. In this situation, an inverted dictionary, or word finder, is necessary.

8.18 Stanaszek, Mary J., et al. *The Inverted Medical Dictionary.* 2d ed. Lancaster, PA, Technomic, 1991.

8.19 Hamilton, Betty and Guidos, Barbara. *The Medical Word Finder: A Reverse Medical Dictionary.* New York, Neal-Schuman, 1987.

8.20 Willeford, George, Jr., comp. *Webster's New World Medical Word Finder.* 4th ed. New York, Prentice-Hall, 1987.

8.21 Lorenzini, Jean A. *Medical Phrase Index.* 2d ed. Oradell, NJ, Medical Economics, 1989.

Both *The Inverted Medical Dictionary* and *The Medical Word Finder* contain an alphabetical list of single words and extended phrases which are likely to be the most obvious to users. Under each heading in *The Inverted Medical Dictionary,* the proper medical term(s) is provided, and in some instances a brief definition is included as well. In addition to the main alphabetical list, this dictionary has sections on eponyms, terms used in prescription writing, drug and chemical abbreviations, and common medical abbreviations. In *The Medical Word Finder,* the entry information for the headings includes technical terminology, synonyms, and, where appropriate, commonly used prefixes and suffixes.

Webster's New World Medical Word Finder was compiled to show health professionals how to spell, syllabicate, divide, and accentuate frequently used medical terms. The book is arranged into ten sections which include a list of prefixes and suffixes; an alphabetical list of tests, arteries, syndromes, etc.; a list of commonly prescribed drugs; and a list of phonetic spellings for 179 problem words.

Lorenzini, a medical transcriber, has taken about 100,000 phrases directly from the medical transcriptions of more than 1,000 physicians and cross-referenced each phrase by each of its main words. *Medical Phrase Index* contains both standard and nonstandard terminology, e.g., barium burger and cafe coronary.

SUBJECT DICTIONARIES

There are numerous dictionaries available that are narrow in scope but expansive in a particular area. Each has features that set it apart from a general medical dictionary.

8.22 Finkel, Asher J., et al. *Current Medical Information and Terminology.* 5th ed. Chicago, American Medical Association, 1981.

8.23 Zwemer, Thomas J. *Boucher's Clinical Dental Terminology.* 4th ed. St. Louis, MO, Mosby, 1993.

8.24 Jablonski, Stanley. *Jablonski's Dictionary of Dentistry.* Reprint edition of *Illustrated Dictionary of Dentistry.* Malabar, FL, Krieger, 1992.

8.25 Miller, Benjamin F. and Keane, Claire B. *Encyclopedia and Dictionary of Medicine, Nursing, and Allied Health.* 5th ed. Philadelphia, PA, Saunders, 1992.

8.26 Glanze, Walter D., ed. *Mosby's Medical, Nursing, and Allied Health Dictionary.* 3d ed. St. Louis, MO, Mosby, 1990. Revised edition of *Mosby's Medical and Nursing Dictionary,* 2d ed., 1986.

Current Medical Information and Terminology is directed toward the individual who must organize medical syndromes and diseases in an orderly system. The alphabetical arrangement, including cross-references, eponyms, and synonyms, leads to the preferred heading for a particular disease. The authors indicate that their system of classification is even suitable for computerization. Each preferred entry includes the term, its code number in the system, and other information including synonyms, etiology, symptoms, physical signs, laboratory data, radiologic findings, pathology, and prognosis. There is a numerical index, an index of diseases by body system, and a section of abbreviations. The book shows how diseases can be categorized for retrieval and statistical purposes.

Dental terminology is often confusing due to the number of specialties and subspecialties in dentistry. *Boucher's* and *Jablonski's* are two dictionaries that provide comprehensive coverage of dental terminology.

Boucher's Current Clinical Dental Terminology is designed for practicing dentists, students, and anyone associated with the delivery of dental care.

Terms from all areas of dentistry are arranged alphabetically; pronunciations and numerous "see" references are included. Topics covered in the appendices include abbreviations, dental etymology, nomenclature, and the official American Dental Association codes for dental procedures.

Jablonski's Illustrated Dictionary of Dentistry attempts to define all terms in all specialties of dentistry and its allied fields. It is arranged in the style of major unabridged medical dictionaries. Definitions are descriptive, include cross-references from secondary to preferred terms, and are supplemented with illustrations and tables. The book contains a guide to dental etymology and appendices that include information on the American Dental Association, the Canadian Dental Association, U.S. and Canadian dental schools, and schools for dental hygiene and dental assisting in the United States.

Miller and Keane's *Encyclopedia and Dictionary* serves as an excellent source for anyone in the allied medical professions because it defines the terminology of those professions. As the title indicates, this book is an encyclopedia and has encyclopedic definitions of entries. As in most dictionaries, entry words are divided by syllables and marked for pronunciation. The book contains good anatomical tables and plates. Its best features are the appendices, which include weights and measures, the 1980 daily dietary allowances, sources of patient education materials, laboratory reference values, and voluntary health and welfare agencies.

Mosby's Medical, Nursing, and Allied Health Dictionary is very encyclopedic in style. It provides sentence definitions and additional material when a definition alone is not sufficient. *Mosby's* is directed to nurses and other health professionals. There are many illustrations and tables, a special 44-page color atlas of human anatomy, and extensive appendices. Unique features of this dictionary include abbreviations and cross-references alphabetized into the text and a print style and size that looks like a textbook instead of a dictionary.

> 8.27 King, Robert C. and Stansfield, William D. *A Dictionary of Genetics.* 4th ed. New York, Oxford University Press, 1990.
> 8.28 Campbell, Robert J. *Psychiatric Dictionary.* 6th ed. New York, Oxford University Press, 1989.
> 8.29 Blauvelt, Carolyn T. and Nelson, Fred R.T. *A Manual of Orthopaedic Terminology.* 5th ed. Chicago, Mosby-Year Book, 1993.

There are literally dozens of specialized subject dictionaries in medically related fields, from chromatography to psychology. These books by King, Campbell, and Blauvelt and Nelson illustrate the diversity that is available as well as the specialized information that may be found in subject dictionaries.

A Dictionary of Genetics includes terms, tables, abbreviations, and molecular formulas from all fields related to genetics. Appendices include a list of periodicals cited in the literature of genetics and a chronology of genetic research and discoveries.

Campbell's *Psychiatric Dictionary* is one of several in this subject area. It contains encyclopedic definitions for many words, extensive cross-references, eponyms, and important names in psychiatry.

A Manual of Orthopaedic Terminology may be used as a general orthopedic dictionary. Terms are classified and arranged into chapters on topics such as the classification of fractures and dislocations, orthopedic tests, signs and maneuvers, prosthetic and surgical intervention, and musculoskeletal research. Several appendices and an extensive index complete the book.

> 8.30 Lawrence, Eleanor, ed. *Henderson's Dictionary of Biological Terms*. 10th ed. New York, Wiley, 1989.
> 8.31 Gray, Peter. *A Dictionary of the Biological Sciences*. Reprint. Malabar, FL, Krieger, 1982.

Dictionaries of biological terms are needed because general medical dictionaries do not provide comprehensive coverage of this terminology that is related to the health sciences. *Henderson's Dictionary* is an alphabetical listing of biological words from all biological and basic medical sciences. A straightforward, uncomplicated, unadorned dictionary, it contains more than 22,500 terms, including transliterated Greek and Russian terms. Plant and animal kingdom classifications (to the order level) are included in the appendices.

A Dictionary of the Biological Sciences is more complicated to use. Major terms, such as chemical terms, are arranged alphabetically, but descriptive terms that require an extended definition are arranged as in a thesaurus. This dictionary includes vernacular terms, several thousand word roots, personal names, and taxa above ordinal rank. Latin and Greek words are anglicized whenever possible. There is also a bibliography of works consulted by the author. Both of these dictionaries are directed at the generalist.

FOREIGN-LANGUAGE DICTIONARIES

There is a need for reference tools that translate a medical term from one language to another. Some definitions of words that are obtained from general dictionaries may not be accurate in the medical context. In addition, more and more health care professionals are treating non-English-speaking patients. The sources described here are examples of foreign-language dictionaries that are available.

8.32 Dorian, A. F., comp. *Elsevier's Encyclopaedic Dictionary of Medicine.* New York, Elsevier, 1988-1990. 4 parts.

8.33 McElroy, Onyria Herrera and Grabb, Lola L. *Spanish-English, English-Spanish Medical Dictionary=Diccionario Médico Español-Inglés, Inglés-Español.* 1st ed. Boston, MA, Little, Brown, 1992.

8.34 Unseld, Dieter Werner. *Medical Dictionary of the English and German Languages: Two Parts in One Volume.* 10th ed., rev. and enl. Stuttgart, Wissenschaftliche Verlagsgesellschaft, 1991.

Elsevier's is available in four separately published parts: general medicine; anatomy; biology, genetics and biochemistry; therapeutic substances. Each title is divided into two sections. The first section is the basic table, which lists the English entries in alphabetical order. Each entry is followed by the English definition and by its French, German, Italian, and Spanish equivalents.

The second section comprises four indexes, one for each language, where the equivalents are listed alphabetically. Each entry in this section has a number which refers to the relevant entry in the basic table.

The *Spanish-English, English-Spanish Medical Dictionary* contains more than 20,000 clearly written entries. The dictionary has sections on common medical abbreviations, simplified grammar in both languages, and conversion tables for translating and interpreting medical terminology. There are three appendices: signs and symptoms of common disorders; lists of phrases used when speaking with patients; and numbers, expressions of time, and weights and measures.

The *Medical Dictionary of the English and German Languages* is divided into two sections: English-German and German-English. The dictionary offers no definitions; only the equivalent term is provided. This source is intended to be useful to not only doctors and dentists, but to pharmacists, chemists, and other medical and life sciences workers.

SYNDROMES, EPONYMS, AND QUOTATIONS

A syndrome is a constant pattern or grouping of abnormal signs or symptoms. Some syndromes have descriptive names and others are eponymic (i.e., named for the individual who first described the syndrome to the medical world). They are important to physicians because they are usually associated with diseases.

8.35 Magalini, Sergio I.; Magalini, Sabina C.; and de Francisci, Giovanni. *Dictionary of Medical Syndromes.* 3d ed. Philadelphia, PA, Lippincott, 1990.

8.36 Durham, Robert H. *Encyclopedia of Medical Syndromes*. New York, Hoeber, 1960.
8.37 Jablonski, Stanley. *Jablonski's Dictionary of Syndromes and Eponymic Diseases*. 2d ed. Malabar, FL, Krieger, 1991.

In terms of information about each syndrome, the *Dictionary of Medical Syndromes* is probably the most comprehensive of the three sources. More than 2,700 syndromes are described, and each explanation includes most of the following information: name of syndrome, synonyms, signs, etiology, pathology, diagnostic procedures, therapy, prognosis, and bibliography. The format is designed for quick reference and is easy to read. Although the text is not cross-referenced, the index is fully cross-referenced to the major headings.

Encyclopedia of Medical Syndromes is not as detailed but it is useful because it covers syndromes not mentioned in *Dictionary of Medical Syndromes*. The syndromes are cross-referenced in the text and indexed by classification (type or organ system). The *Encyclopedia* contains references to literature that elaborates on or clarifies the syndromes.

A typical entry in *Jablonski's Dictionary of Syndromes and Eponymic Diseases* begins with the name of the person for whom the syndrome or condition is named, the eponym, its synonyms, and the definition. The entries include a bibliography or references to recent literature and the original report of the syndrome or disease. Synonyms are listed separately. When helpful, illustrations are used.

8.38 Strauss, Maurice B. *Familiar Medical Quotations*. Boston, MA, Little, Brown, 1968.
8.39 Daintith, John and Isaacs, Amanda. *Medical Quotes: A Thematic Dictionary*. New York, Facts on File, 1989.
8.40 Kelly, Emerson Crosby. *Encyclopedia of Medical Sources*. Baltimore, MD, Williams & Wilkins, 1948.

Important statements have been made by all types of people about medicine, disease, health care, and other health-related subjects. Strauss has brought together more than 7,000 such comments in *Familiar Medical Quotations*. The quotations are arranged alphabetically by category and chronologically within categories. The index, an alphabetical listing of keywords from the quotations, gives general access to the quotations. The book is authoritative—nearly all quotations have been verified. A secondary source is usually given if a quotation could not be verified. *Familiar Medical Quotations* is a compendium of who said what in the health sciences.

Medical Quotes: A Thematic Dictionary is a collection of remarks, writings, and sayings about medical and related subjects. Quotations are arranged under theme headings of general interest. Within each theme section, the quotations are in alphabetical order by author's last name. Entry information includes the author's name, dates, a short biography, and a source reference for the quotation. Cross-references are provided to related topics. Two indexes—keyword-key phrase and author—provide access to the quotations. The reference in the index is to the theme and to the number of the quote within that theme.

The title of Kelly's work, *Encyclopedia of Medical Sources*, is somewhat misleading. The book is a list of more than 6,000 names and the medical discoveries attributed to those individuals. It includes anatomical points of reference, operations, tests, treatments, diseases, important writings, and the source of publication of the discovery. The book is fully cross-referenced. Rather than listing individual names, the index lists the anatomical parts, tests, diseases, and so on.

CHAPTER 9

Handbooks and Manuals

Fred W. Roper

Handbooks and manuals are compendia of vast amounts of information on a variety of topics and are useful in answering the so-called "factual" question. These publications are of prime importance to the researcher in the health sciences. Grogan states that "a library with no more than a sound collection of handbooks can answer 90 percent of quick-reference queries" [1]. The practical nature of the information contained in handbooks and manuals assists the researcher or clinician in day-to-day work. Handbooks and manuals range in format from one-volume data books to multivolume compendia, which may be encyclopedic in nature. This chapter discusses three types of handbooks and manuals: data books; laboratory compendia; and handbooks relating to diagnosis, classification, and physiology.

> 9.1 Powell, Russell H., ed. *Handbooks and Tables in Science and Technology.* 2d ed. Phoenix, AZ, Oryx Press, 1983.

Powell has provided a comprehensive guide to a variety of reference materials in *Handbooks and Tables in Science and Technology.* All areas of science and technology are covered, including the biological and health sciences. Although the emphasis is on English-language materials, important works from around the world are included. The critical annotations enable users to determine whether or not the work cited contains the required information.

DATA BOOKS

Data books present basic scientific information in a concise format. Tables, such as the properties of substances, mathematical data, boiling points, and toxicities, are often used in the presentation of the data and are sometimes accompanied by text. Frequent revision is necessary to assure that the material presented is up to date. The key to successful use of a data book is an adequate and detailed index.

9.2 Altman, Philip, and Dittmer, Dorothy, eds. *Biology Data Book*. 3d ed. Bethesda, MD, Federation of American Societies for Experimental Biology, 1972-1974. 3 vols.

9.3 Altman, Philip, and Dittmer, Dorothy, eds. *Growth, Including Reproduction and Morphological Development*. Washington, DC, Federation of American Societies for Experimental Biology, 1962.

9.4 Altman, Philip, and Katz, Dorothy, eds. *Human Health and Disease*. Bethesda, MD, Federation of American Societies for Experimental Biology, 1977.

These important publications from the Federation of American Societies for Experimental Biology (FASEB) are based on contributions from a large number of research scientists.

The *Biology Data Book* is intended to serve as a basic reference in the field of biology. With broadened scope and coverage in the third edition, the revised publication appears in three volumes: Volume 1, genetics and cytology, reproduction, development, and growth; Volume 2, biological regulators and toxins, environment and survival, and parasitism; and Volume 3, nutrition, digestion and excretion, metabolism, respiration and circulation, and blood and other body fluids. Each volume is indexed independently. An important feature is the inclusion of references for the sources of the data. Coverage is restricted "to man and the more important laboratory, domestic, commercial, and field organisms" (Preface). Even so, many species are included.

Growth, Including Reproduction and Morphological Development is an example of the specialized handbooks that have been produced under the auspices of FASEB. Similar in format to the *Biology Data Book*, it is a compendium that presents data on various aspects of normal growth. The most recent title in the series of biological handbooks is *Human Health and Disease*. The seven sections of the handbook present data in the form of 186 tables of quantitative and descriptive data. Contributors are identified and the series continues to include citations to the literature.

9.5 Lentner, C., ed. *Geigy Scientific Tables*. 8th rev. and enl. ed. Basle, Switzerland, Ciba-Geigy, 1981- .

The goal of *Geigy Scientific Tables* is to provide doctors and scientists with concise compendia of data on a variety of topics. The book is a continuing publication that is divided into individual volumes. This makes it possible to incorporate additional chapters and helps ensure that the information is current. Literature references to the sources of data are a part of each presentation. The six volumes published to date provide coverage of body fluids, statistical tables, physical chemistry, biochemistry, the heart, and bacteria.

9.6 Lide, David R., ed. *CRC Handbook of Chemistry and Physics.* 74th ed. Boca Raton, FL, CRC Press, 1993/1994.
9.7 Fasman, Gerald D., ed. *Practical Handbook of Biochemistry and Molecular Biology.* Boca Raton, FL, CRC Press, 1989.
9.8 *Composite Index for CRC Handbooks.* 3d ed. Boca Raton, FL, CRC Press, 1991. 3 vols. *Supplement.* Boca Raton, FL, CRC Press, 1992.

An important group of handbooks is published by the CRC Press. The tremendous growth of scientific knowledge in the 20th century has led to the expansion of titles since the first title, *CRC Handbook of Chemistry and Physics,* appeared in 1913. Now numbering more than fifty titles, the series is intended to provide coverage of many subject areas in the sciences. Titles in the series range from broad areas such as chemistry and physics to specialized topics such as chemical laboratory science, hospital safety, and applied optics.

The 74th edition of *CRC Handbook of Chemistry and Physics* aims to provide broad coverage of all types of information frequently needed by physical scientists. References are provided to guide users to other compilations and databases if the *Handbook* does not have the answer.

With the increase of available data and the ever-growing interdisciplinary nature of science, the CRC Handbook series has expanded to meet reference requirements of the newer disciplines through the development of comprehensive multivolume handbooks. The *Handbook of Biochemistry and Molecular Biology* effectively demonstrates this concept. The third edition (1975-1977) is published in nine volumes that cover proteins; nucleic acids; lipids, carbohydrates, and steroids; and physical and chemical data. This multivolume title has been updated by the *Practical Handbook of Biochemistry and Molecular Biology.* It is a single-volume handbook designed for easy use in the laboratory.

To provide a master key to the material contained in the CRC handbooks, the *Composite Index* has been published. Information and data included in several of the handbooks or a single volume of a particular title may be of value to the user. However, to access the material the user must check the index of each volume. To assist in the gathering of data that may be contained in the various titles, the *Composite Index for CRC Handbooks* alphabetically merges the individual volume indexes into a three-part index and provides the volume and page number for each entry. The

Composite Index and *Supplement*—also available on a single CD-ROM—offer access to the contents of 368 handbook volumes. CRC Press plans to issue the *Composite Index* annually beginning in 1994.

> 9.9 *Report of the Task Group on Reference Man.* Reprint. Report No. 23, International Commission on Radiological Protection. New York, Pergamon, 1992.

Although the report was prepared to assist in studies on the effects of radiation on humans, the data that have been included cause it to have broad application. The compilers limited their attention to those characteristics of humans "which are known to be important or which are likely to be significant for estimation of dose from sources of radiation within or outside the body" (Introduction). Even with this limitation, the book serves as an important complement to the handbooks discussed above.

LABORATORY COMPENDIA

These materials serve both an encyclopedia and a textbook function. They generally consist of essays relating to techniques, methodology, interpretation, and analysis used in diagnosis. Representative examples include:

> 9.10 Henry, John B., ed. *Clinical Diagnosis and Management by Laboratory Methods.* 18th ed. Philadelphia, PA, Saunders, 1991.
> 9.11 Tilton, Richard C., et al. *Clinical Laboratory Medicine.* St. Louis, MO, Mosby-Year Book, 1992.
> 9.12 *Methods in Enzymology.* New York, Academic Press. Vol. 1- , 1955- . Annual.

Clinical Diagnosis and Management by Laboratory Methods is a comprehensive textbook that emphasizes molecular and clinical pathology. Information is presented through a series of essays and is organized by subject: the clinical laboratory, clinical chemistry, medical microscopy, hematology and coagulation, immunology and immunopathology, medical microbiology, and administration of the clinical laboratory.

Clinical Laboratory Medicine discusses the rationale for ordering tests, interpreting results, and basic pathophysiology of numerous disease states. It also provides detailed descriptions of all laboratory procedures.

Both titles are composite works that have been prepared through the collaboration of a large number of experts in the various fields represented. Illustrations, tables, and color plates supplement the material in the essays. Bibliographic references provide information on the sources of the material presented, as well as additional reading for the student in the field.

Specialized works in laboratory analysis abound, and *Methods of Enzymology* represents this type of publication. Each volume (or group of volumes) in the series concentrates on a particular topic, with an editor and a group of contributors providing essays on a state-of-the-art approach. Other continuing serial publications carry out the same objectives for their particular specialized areas.

HANDBOOKS RELATED TO DIAGNOSIS AND CLASSIFICATION

Nomenclature is defined by *Webster's Third New International Dictionary* as "a system or set of names or designations used in a particular science, discipline, or art and formally adopted or sanctioned by the usage of its practitioners." In medicine and its related fields there are a number of works that set out a systematic terminology for a particular purpose.

9.13 *CPT 1994, Physician's Current Procedural Terminology.* 4th ed., rev. Chicago, American Medical Association, 1993.

9.14 International Union of Biochemistry and Molecular Biology. Nomenclature Committee. *Enzyme Nomenclature 1992: Recommendations of the Nomenclature Committee of the International Union of Biochemistry and Molecular Biology.* San Diego, Published for the International Union of Biochemistry and Molecular Biology by Academic Press, 1992.

9.15 *Manual of the International Statistical Classification of Diseases, Injuries, and Causes of Death.* 9th rev. Geneva, Switzerland, World Health Organization, 1977. 2 vols.

9.16 *The International Classification of Diseases, 9th Revision, Clinical Modification: ICD-9-CM.* 4th ed. Washington, DC, U.S. Department of Health and Human Services, Public Health Service, Health Care Financing Administration, 1991. 2 vols.

9.17 *Diagnostic and Statistical Manual of Mental Disorders: DSM-III-R.* 3d ed., rev. Washington, DC, American Psychiatric Association, 1987. *DSM-IV Draft Criteria.* Washington, DC, The Association, 1993.

9.18 Berkow, Robert, ed. *The Merck Manual of Diagnosis and Therapy.* 16th ed. Rahway, NJ, Merck, 1992.

The purpose of *CPT 1994* is to provide a standardized listing of terms and codes for reporting medical services and procedures performed by physicians. The terms, arranged by body system, are each assigned a five-digit code. Access to individual codes is provided through an alphabetical index arranged by procedure, anatomical site, condition, synonyms, abbreviations, and eponyms.

Enzyme Nomenclature 1992 is an example of a standardized terminology created to bring order to a particular field. This book is based on the recommendations of the nomenclature committee of the International Union of Biochemistry and Molecular Biology. It was created to organize the chaos that existed in the 1950s when many new enzymes were being discovered and named haphazardly. *Enzyme Nomenclature* includes the names of more than 3,196 enzymes and a detailed mechanism that is used in naming new enzymes.

The *Manual of the International Statistical Classification of Diseases, Injuries, and Causes of Death* represents "a system of categories to which morbid entities are assigned according to some established criteria" (Introduction). These categories make it possible for standardization of the collection of data related to diseases, injuries, and causes of death. To facilitate the study of disease, the scheme has been arranged so that each specific disease entity has "a separate title in the classification only when its separation is war-ranted because the frequency of its occurrence, or its importance as a morbid condition, justifies its isolation as a separate category" (Introduc-tion). This element of grouping represents the difference between a classi-fication for statistical purposes and a nomenclature that must be as detailed as possible to provide for all possible names.

The International Classification of Diseases (ICD-9) is a decimal classifica-tion system. The three digits preceding the decimal represent the chosen categories in seventeen broad areas; digits following the decimal represent the specific diseases found in each category. (Although volume 1 [Tabular List] of *ICD-10* was published in 1992, volume 2 [Instruction Manual] and volume 3 [Alphabetical Index] are not yet available. The federal govern-ment anticipates using the 10th revision, but not before the year 2000.)

ICD-9-CM is the U.S. adaptation of *ICD-9*. The clinical modification provides a common classification of diseases and related entities to be used by all agencies and institutions. The intent of *ICD-9-CM* is "to serve as a useful tool in the area of classification of morbidity data for indexing of medical records, medical care review, and ambulatory and other medical care programs, as well as for basic health statistics" (Foreword). The mod-ification provides the greater precision that is required for the maintenance of clinical records.

A complementary publication, *Diagnostic and Statistical Manual of Mental Disorders: DSM-III-R*, is based on the mental disorders section in *The Inter-national Classification of Diseases*. The *DSM-III-R* provides information on nomenclature and specific criteria as guidelines for making each diagnosis. (*DSM-IV* should be available by early 1994.)

The *Merck Manual of Diagnosis and Therapy* contains discussions of factors related to rational diagnostic reasoning and effective therapy, including discussions of symptoms and signs. The twenty-three sections are subdivided into chapters that go into considerable detail. The work attempts to serve as a reference guide for the whole range of medical disorders.

Handbooks and manuals are likely to be used heavily in ready reference because of the diverse information they contain. The titles presented in this chapter are but a few of the possible sources that could have been included. Many are standard titles that should be found in all health sciences libraries; others represent the variety that is available.

REFERENCE

1. Grogan D. Science and technology: an introduction to the literature. 4th ed., rev. London: Clive Bingley, 1982:73.

CHAPTER 10

Drug Information Sources

Diane L. Fishman

Drug information is a broad field covering all aspects of the actions of drugs and chemicals on living systems. It includes the traditional fields of pharmacology (the study of the physiological actions of drugs), pharmacy (the compounding, manufacture, and dispensing of drugs), and toxicology (the study of hazardous effects of chemicals). Increasingly, pharmacists are focusing on "pharmaceutical care" (advising customers on the proper use of drugs).

Drug information questions are directed to librarians from a number of sources. A physician may want to know if a particular symptom or side effect has previously been associated with the administration of a particular drug. An occupational health specialist may ask if there is a relationship between a clinical symptom and daily exposure to a chemical in the work environment. A pharmacist may need the American equivalent of a drug prescribed in a foreign country. A nurse may want more information about a drug being administered to a patient to assist in monitoring the patient's response to the drug. Members of the public frequently ask questions about drugs they are taking or about additives in the food they eat.

The proliferation of therapeutic drugs is a relatively recent phenomenon. The earliest therapeutic agents were primarily plant and animal substances, and mentioned in early materia medica are such things as garlic, juniper berries, and dragon's blood (of plant origin); these were administered usually as extracts, poultices, or powders. Still in use today are drugs from some of these plant sources—for example, digitalis is obtained from foxglove and morphine from the opium poppy. Significant advances in organic chemistry provided for the chemical isolation of these therapeutic agents from the plant and animal sources.

Since World War II, the drug industry has grown tremendously. The combination of advanced techniques in chemical synthesis and a better understanding of the underlying causes of diseases resulted in many therapeutic agents becoming available. A quick comparison of editions of the *Physicians' Desk Reference (PDR)* (*see* 10.11)—a guide to drugs for the physician—from the late 1940s with those published today shows dramatic differences. The early editions list such agents as estrogenic substance in oil, liver injection, and desiccated kidney of hogs, while recent editions list very specific chemical entities. The size of the *PDR* has also greatly increased; the current edition is more than fifteen times larger than the first, suggesting a substantial increase in the number of drugs available and in the information about them. The increasing use of drugs has even resulted in a new field—iatrogenic disease—meaning "physician-induced disease," referring primarily to clinical problems resulting from the use of therapeutic drugs.

Information about drugs is complex due to government regulation. The Food and Drug Administration (FDA) regulates all drugs in interstate commerce and is responsible for overseeing the labeling of drugs and ensuring that they are both safe and effective. These regulations are published in the *Code of Federal Regulations, Title 21: Food and Drugs* (available electronically as 21 CFR on BRS). The FDA requires the pharmaceutical company to notify prescribing physicians of contraindications (i.e., when not to use a drug), warnings, and adverse effects of drugs. Increasingly they are being asked to provide more information on the drug package label. In recent years, the Occupational Safety and Health Administration (OSHA) has become more involved in monitoring the effects of chemicals in industrial settings.

The federal government has established strict regulations regarding the introduction of new drugs and the monitoring of drugs already available. When a pharmaceutical company has a chemical entity that it believes has significant therapeutic value, it files an Investigational New Drug Application (IND) with the FDA. The drug company must then conduct documented studies to demonstrate the therapeutic value and safety of the drug. After substantial testing in animals, the IND testing begins in very small groups of healthy human (usually male) volunteers (Phase I studies) to determine safety. Next, clinical trials are expanded to include a small group of human subjects suffering from the disease the drug is intended to treat (Phase II studies). These studies continue to review safety as well as efficacy. If these trials are satisfactory, the study moves into Phase III, where the drug is given to a larger and more diverse population. When sufficient data have been collected, the pharmaceutical company submits another application to the FDA, a New Drug Application (NDA), with its data on the safety and effectiveness of the drug. Approval of the NDA means that the drug is approved for marketing and can be prescribed by licensed practitioners within the prescribing laws of the Comprehensive Drug Act of 1970. Prior to this approval, the drug may be used only by certain physicians who have been approved to handle investigational drugs. As the drug is made available to potentially millions of patients, additional side effects may show up. For instance, it is generally only at this point that pregnant women will have access to the drug (prior tests for dangers to the fetus are performed on animals). Therefore, studies continue under Phase IV to cover postmarketing surveillance.

Information on the drug in its preclinical stages, especially before it is patented, may be difficult to obtain. Studies usually appear first in the chemical literature (or the biological literature if it is a naturally derived substance). The biological literature is also a good place to search for early toxicity or carcinogenicity animal studies performed before the IND is submitted. Unfortunately, the NDA with its documented evidence never becomes a part of the public domain. It is considered to be proprietary information available only to the company and the FDA. However, researchers often publish their experiences with the drug during clinical trials. This material is retrievable through the journal and report literature.

After the patent on a drug expires, other companies may wish to market a generic equivalent. These companies need only submit an Abbreviated New Drug Application (ANDA) to show 80% bioequivalency; that is, when administered in the same amounts, the equivalent drug will provide at least 80% of the same biological or physiological availability. Applications for biotechnology products undergo a similar review process known as the Product License Application (PLA).

GUIDES TO THE LITERATURE

10.1 Snow, Bonnie. *Drug Information; A Guide to Current Resources*. Chicago, Medical Library Association, 1989.
10.2 Andrews, Theodora. *Guide to the Literature of Pharmacy and the Pharmaceutical Sciences*. Littleton, CO, Libraries Unlimited, 1986.
10.3 Sewell, Winifred. *Guide to Drug Information*. Hamilton, IL, Drug Intelligence Publications, 1976.

Guides can help the beginning librarian put the drug literature into perspective. In addition, they can suggest additional sources or works in specialized areas which librarians at any level may wish to consult. For instance, Snow's *Drug Information* is a very helpful guide that goes into greater depth than this chapter. The volume provides background on drug nomenclature, pharmaceutic law, and the evaluation of drug information sources in addition to descriptions of particular reference works. Andrews' *Guide* is a larger work with a bibliographic emphasis. Because Andrews focuses primarily on the description of specific sources, the book covers reference tools not mentioned in the Snow book. The third source, Sewell's *Guide to Drug Information,* has now become dated, although a new edition is in the planning stages. In the meantime, the background information and many comparative tables in the original edition remain useful.

DRUG NOMENCLATURE

One of the major problems in using the drug literature is recognizing the multiplicity of names for a given chemical compound and understanding how reference sources must be approached depending on the type of name. A thorough understanding of these names is essential (Figure 10-1). When a pharmaceutical company is investigating a large number of chemicals for possible therapeutic activity, it frequently assigns alphanumeric designations or code names. Often, a code name is the first designation in the primary literature.

Similarly, the Chemical Abstract Service provides a separate registry number for each chemical compound (including drugs). One thing to remember about the registry number is that European countries commonly name the drug for the parent compound. In the United States, it is more usual to use the salt form (the compound formulated as a salt so that it will dissolve more easily in water), which will generally have a different registry number. Because indexes vary on whether the parent or salt registry number is used, the experienced searcher should try to identify both registry numbers for full retrieval.

The chemical name describes the chemical structure of a drug. There are a number of conventions for these chemical names, which are often very lengthy. Consequently, there is a need for a shorter, "common" name to describe a drug. "Aspirin" and "tetracycline" are examples of these more easily handled names. Common names are also called "generic" or "nonproprietary" names. Names used by a manufacturer to describe specific marketed products are called "trade," "proprietary," or "brand" names. Trade names are registered trademarks, as are the color, shape, and markings of each pill or capsule. Two or more manufacturers may market the same generic drug, but each may also have its own trade name representing its specific product. These products may differ; although the active ingredients are the same, each manufacturer may use different ingredients in compounding the drug or in holding it together. The composition of a pill, other than amounts of active ingredients, is a proprietary or trade secret, but is often available from the manufacturer if a patient has a reaction to the medication. Inactive ingredients are also sometimes listed in resources such as POISINDEX in Micromedex's Computerized Clinical Information System (CCIS) (*see* 10.40) and *AHFS Drug Information* (*see* 10.14).

Figure 10-1. Types of Drug Names

Research code names:	Ro 5-0690 NSC-115748
CAS registry number:	438-41-5
Chemical name:	3H-1, 4-Benzodiazepin-2-amine, 7-chloro-N-methyl-5-phenyl, 4-oxide, monohydrochloride
Generic name:	Chlordiazepoxide hydrochloride
Official name:	Chlordiazepoxide hydrochloride
Trade names:	Librium (Hoffman-LaRoche) SK-Lygen (Smith, Kline and French)
Molecular formula:	$C_{16}H_{14}ClN_3O,HCL$

Structural formula:

Another source of confusion is the multiplicity of generic names. Two companies working with the same drug may call it by different generic names. In the past, this practice has led to such confusion that now "official" generic names are designated. The United States Adopted Names (USAN) Commission has the authority to declare a specific generic name as the officially recognized common name, the "adopted name," in the United States. If another company wants to market a preparation of that drug, it will use this "official" generic name.

The nomenclature problem is compounded on an international scale. Other countries also have authorized bodies to establish official names; the World Health Organization's *International Nonproprietary Names* attempts to unify official names in all participating countries, but differences still exist. Furthermore, because of the strict laws regulating investigational drugs in this country, new drugs are often available much sooner elsewhere.

These variations in nomenclature cause a range of difficulties. For instance, a patient having been prescribed a French drug travels to the United States and needs a refill of an American equivalent. A British doctor, taking an American medical licensure exam, finds "meperidine" on the examination questions rather than "pethidine," the name to which British doctors are accustomed. Researchers may read a German article about the anticoagulant "ancrod" and want to know if there is an American equivalent.

The librarian must understand the many types of names to use literature sources effectively. Some publications, particularly those originating from commercial sources, may be arranged by proprietary or trade name. Others, especially those from professional associations, are usually arranged by nonproprietary or generic name. Books published in other countries use their own official generic names, which are sometimes different from the American form. Some sources are limited to prescription drugs, while others include nonprescription (over the counter or OTC) medications. The librarian, presented with a drug name, may not immediately know what type of name it is. The first step is to determine the type of name and then go to appropriate reference sources.

SOURCES OF DRUG IDENTIFICATION

A number of sources should be readily available for finding brief information about drugs, particularly for identifying trade and generic names.

10.4 *American Drug Index*. Philadelphia, Lippincott, 1956- . Annual.

10.5 *USAN and the USP Dictionary of Drug Names.* Rockville, MD, United States Pharmacopoeial Convention, 1961/71- . Annual.

10.6 *The Merck Index: An Encyclopedia of Chemicals, Drugs, and Biologicals.* 11th ed. Rahway, NJ, Merck, 1989.

10.7 *Unlisted Drugs*. New York, Pharmaceutical Division, Special Libraries Association, Vol. 1- , 1949- . Monthly. *Unlisted Drugs Index
Guide/9*. Chatham, NJ, Unlisted Drugs, 1992.

The *American Drug Index (ADI)* includes brief information on a large
number of drugs; its comprehensive coverage in one alphabet of over-the-
counter and prescription drugs by both trade and generic names makes it
an ideal source for initial consultation. Trade name entries include
manufacturer's name, generic or chemical names, composition and
strength, pharmaceutical forms available, package size, dosage, and a brief
indication of use. Generic name entries frequently include an indication of
whether the name is listed in the *U.S. Pharmacopeia (USP)* (*see* 10.18) or
National Formulary (NF) (*see* 10.18), USAN (U.S. Adopted Name) (*see* 10.5),
or BAN (British Adopted Name). Generic name entries provide a brief
description of use and also list proprietary products that include the drug.
Trade names are given for combination drugs—products that contain more
than one therapeutic agent. The *ADI* also provides addresses and phone
numbers of distributors and contains other useful appendices such as a list
of oral dosage forms that should not be crushed.

Another primary source for brief drug information is the *USAN and the
USP Dictionary of Drug Names*. This compilation lists the United States
Adopted Names selected and released since June 15, 1961. For each USAN,
the following information is provided: year published as a USAN, a pronunciation guide, molecular formula, chemical name, Chemical Abstracts
Services (CAS) registry number, pharmacological or therapeutic activity
claim, brand names under which the drug is marketed, manufacturer or
distributor, and the structural formula. The *USAN and the USP Dictionary
of Drug Names* is particularly useful for its inclusion of earlier drug names.
An excellent introduction details the purpose and history of the USAN
Council and procedures which establish a USAN. Appendices include a
cumulative list of drugs or biologicals which have been granted "orphan
status." For these substances, federal legislation mandates that the developing company have exclusive marketing rights to recoup its investment
because the product has theoretically been developed for a small market of
individuals suffering from a rare disease. There are also indexes by CAS
registry number or NSC number. Caution is required, however. A listing in
the *USAN and the USP* does not indicate that the drug is marketed in this
country; it only means that an official name has been designated. Drugs not
currently available in the United States are listed under their International
Nonproprietary Names (INN). In addition, even if the USAN is given, it is
wise to remember that U.S. drugs are typically named about the time they
are patented and go into clinical trials. Many years may pass until the drug
receives final approval for marketing.

A source of brief information about all types of chemicals, including drugs, is *Merck Index*. When this publication began in 1889, it was only a list of products marketed by the Merck Company. Now in its 11th edition, *Merck Index* has evolved into a comprehensive encyclopedia of chemicals, drugs, and biological substances. *Merck Index* must be accessed through its index, because cross-references do not exist in the body of the work. In addition to standard information such as chemical name, structural formula, and brief description of use, *Merck Index* includes references to patents and journal articles describing the preparation of the chemical. Rounding out this work's utility as a general reference source, there is an index by molecular formula and several appendices, including a listing of organic named reactions, tables of radioactive isotopes, mathematical tables, and tables that correlate the CAS registry number and the substance name. One table lists monographs deleted from the last two editions, a reminder that librarians should not hastily discard older versions of this title.

A unique tool in the drug literature is a serial publication called *Unlisted Drugs*. Begun in 1949 by the Pharmaceutical Division of the Special Libraries Association, this publication was designed to bridge the gap between standard reference textbooks and reports of new drugs in the periodical literature. Drugs are considered "unlisted" when they are not included in several major works such as *American Drug Index* or *Merck Index*, which are referred to by the producers of *Unlisted Drugs* as "exclusion sources." Currently the exclusion sources for *Unlisted Drugs* are the latest editions of *American Drug Index* (10.4); *Merck Index* (10.6); *Martindale: The Extra Pharmacopoeia*, (10.9); *Rote Liste*, a listing of drug products marketed in Germany; *Vidal Dictionnaire*, a listing of French-marketed products; and all previous issues of *Unlisted Drugs*.

Unlisted Drugs provides only brief information on each drug, including composition, manufacturer, pharmacological action, and a literature citation. It may or may not give the structural formula for a drug but provides excellent coverage for research code names and includes equivalent forms when available. *Unlisted Drugs* is also available in card format.

Another feature of *Unlisted Drugs* is its excellent book review section. New books from around the world are listed and summarized. As an adjunct service, *Unlisted Drugs* offers a book ordering service so that smaller libraries do not have to deal directly with individual publishers to obtain the materials. A core reference collection in drug nomenclature might include *Unlisted Drugs* and its exclusion sources.

The *Unlisted Drugs Index Guide* cumulates all entries since the first volume and is now in its ninth edition covering 1949 through 1991. A separate index by drug number is included. Beginning in 1968, combination drugs are indexed under each active ingredient. Trade names are capitalized to distinguish them from generic names. Index coding can be somewhat bewildering but symbols are explained in detail in the introduction. Overall, the index contains more than 210,000 entries, making it an excellent source for both old and new drugs.

COMPREHENSIVE TREATISES AND TEXTBOOKS

The sources mentioned in the previous section do not give extensive information about drugs, but they do identify whether a drug name is trade or generic and give some indication of the manufacturer of a drug. Armed with this brief information, the librarian may next wish to consult a more comprehensive source, which usually will give a detailed description of the drug's pharmacological action.

10.8 Gilman, Alfred, and Goodman, Louis S. *Goodman and Gilman's The Pharmacological Basis of Therapeutics.* 8th ed. Elmsford, NY, Pergamon, 1990.

10.9 *Martindale: The Extra Pharmacopoeia.* 30th ed. London, Pharmaceutical Press, 1993.

10.10 Gennaro, Alfonso R., ed. *Remington's Pharmaceutical Sciences.* 18th ed. Easton, PA, Mack, 1990.

Goodman and Gilman's The Pharmacological Basis of Therapeutics has long been considered the "blue bible of pharmacology." It has been a standard textbook in medical and pharmacy schools and is an extremely valuable treatise of drug information. The first chapter is concerned with general principles, after which chapters are arranged by mode of action—for example, drugs acting on the central nervous system, anesthetics, and cardiovascular drugs. Drugs with a long history of use, such as curare, morphine, and penicillin, have brief histories. The bulk of the material, however, relates to pharmacologic action, with emphasis placed on comparisons of similarly acting drugs.

Martindale: The Extra Pharmacopoeia provides similar, comprehensive information and is also arranged by drug classes. Each drug monograph is lengthy, including pharmacological action and adverse effects. Because regulations regarding new drugs are not as stringent in other countries as they are in the United States, *Martindale's* international coverage includes many drugs not available here, as well as providing foreign equivalents of drugs that are marketed in this country. Because this is a British publication, the monographs are listed under British Adopted Names, but other official names, including USANs, are given immediately thereafter when available. Following each monograph is an extensive bibliography and a listing of proprietary forms, identifying the marketed names and countries of origin.

An index correlates all generic and trade names. *Martindale* is also available online full text through DIALOG and as a module of Micromedex's Computerized Clinical Information System (CCIS) (*see* 10.40). Although the print version is only updated approximately every five years, the electronic versions are revised annually.

The third source, *Remington's Pharmaceutical Sciences,* provides extensive information from a pharmaceutical viewpoint. Used as a textbook by many pharmacy schools, *Remington's* includes information on specific drugs, drug preparation and delivery, the practice of pharmacy, and pharmacy laws (for example, the Comprehensive Drug Act of 1970).

COMMERCIAL SOURCES OF DRUG INFORMATION

There are a number of sources that give information about specific market products. The pharmaceutical manufacturer is responsible for providing certain basic information, the content of which is approved by the FDA. One mechanism by which the manufacturer informs the physician about a specific product is the "package insert," a brief brochure that generally includes the trade and chemical names; pharmacological action; indications and contraindications; warnings, precautions, and adverse reactions; dosage and overdosage; dosage forms; and, in most cases, references. The package insert is not necessarily complete or balanced. Although the FDA has agreed to the manufacturer's statements about the product and the manufacturer is legally responsible for the accuracy of information included, the package insert remains a publicity and promotion mechanism for the manufacturer. A package insert does not compare or evaluate a given drug with other agents.

> 10.11 *Physicians' Desk Reference.* Montvale, NJ, Medical Economics, 1947- . Annual.
>
> 10.12 *Drug Facts and Comparisons.* St. Louis, MO, Facts and Comparisons, Lippincott, 1945- . Loose-leaf, annual hardcopy edition; monthly updates available in loose-leaf or microfiche. Formerly: *Facts and Comparisons.*
>
> 10.13 *Physicians' GenRx 1993.* Smithtown, NY, Data Pharmaceutica, 1993. Formerly: *Physicians' Generix.*

Package inserts are collected and published annually in the *Physicians' Desk Reference,* popularly known as the *PDR*. Information in the *PDR* is arranged by company name and lists many, but not all, products marketed in the United States. It is particularly useful for dosage, composition of each product, contraindications, warnings, use, and adverse effects. Indexes are by brand name; type of action or preparation; and generic, chemical, and manufacturer's name. Also included is a picture section of the most frequently marketed products. The physical representation of capsules and tablets is registered for each manufacturer, just as the names are trademarked. Unfortunately, the color palette is not always accurate. In addition, pictures are arranged by manufacturer, which makes it difficult, although not impossible, to use this source to identify pills or tablets in unmarked containers. (Better sources are the electronic database IDENTIDEX, offered as part of Micromedex's Computerized Clinical Information System [*see* 10.40], or *USP DI v. 2 Advice to the Patient* [*see* 10.34].) Because the *PDR* is a source of manufacturer disclaimer, side effects are enumerated in great detail, although there is often no indication of the severity or frequency of the side effects. For example, because the manufacturing industry cannot conduct safety tests in pregnant humans, the work is liberally peppered with the statement, "safety of this drug during pregnancy is unknown."

The earliest editions of the *PDR* carried the subtitle "for the physician's desk only," and volumes are still often distributed free to physicians as a marketing tool. However, with the recent consumer movement in health care, this statement has been removed, and the *PDR* is now for sale throughout the country in bookstores serving the general public. Many health care consumers regularly ask health sciences librarians for the *PDR*, and the public's reliance on this tool should be a topic of general concern to librarians. First, the information is not necessarily unbiased but represents only what the FDA has approved the manufacturer to say. Second, the coverage is selective, as drug companies are charged for inclusion. Therefore, not all drug companies participate, and those that do typically only include their more profitable drugs. Third, librarians should understand that the information included about drug use is not necessarily complete. Physicians can legally prescribe drugs for therapeutic applications which have not yet been approved by the FDA, and these unlabelled uses will not generally be addressed in the *PDR*. Finally, the information in the *PDR* is written in technical language and may be difficult for the general public to understand. Because rare side effects are included, the work may prove unnecessarily frightening to the nonprofessional. Perhaps one of the greatest challenges to the health sciences librarian is to channel members of the public from the *PDR* to more appropriate sources.

The success of the *PDR* has encouraged a number of spin-offs. Some, like the *PDR for Nonprescription Drugs*, cover a drug category. Because the *PDR* itself includes over-the-counter drugs, there is a good deal of overlap. However, the *PDR for Nonprescription Drugs* does include some drugs not discussed in the *PDR* so that it complements rather than duplicates the more well-known volume. Another *PDR* product, the *PDR Guide to Drug Interactions, Side Effects Indications* (*see* 10.29) does not really stand alone but acts as a combined index to the *PDR*, *PDR for Nonprescription Drugs*, and

PDR for Ophthalmology. The *PDR Family Guide to Prescription Drugs* is a new title aimed at the lay public. *PDR* volumes are usually updated annually.

Drug Facts and Comparisons is a comprehensive compendium of drug information that is heavily used by pharmacists. It is available both in loose-leaf and as an annual bound volume; the monthly updates are available in loose-leaf or microfiche. The evaluative monographs are based on FDA material as well as journal articles and report literature. The work is arranged by therapeutic classification to facilitate comparisons of drugs. For each drug or class of drugs, the following information is given: actions, indications, contraindications, warnings and precautions, drug interactions, adverse reactions, overdosage, patient information, and administration and dosage. Unlabelled uses of drugs are included. Many tables compare drugs within each class and include a comparison of relative costs. This is a useful source for its currency and for its inclusion of both prescription and nonprescription medications.

Formerly entitled *Physicians' Generix* and now in its third year of publication, the *Physicians' GenRx* covers all prescribing information on FDA approved pharmaceuticals. Although it includes drugs for which there is no generic equivalent, it is most useful for comparisons of generic drugs and their alternatives. Often omitted from drug handbooks, compound drugs are here, grouped by substances contained so that, for instance, all medications which contain belladonna, kaolin, paregoric, and pectin (Donnagel-PG, Kaopectolin-PG, etc.) can be reviewed together. The work includes average wholesale prices (an especially useful feature), therapeutic equivalences (drugs that can be substituted for one another), approval and patent dates, HCFA reimbusement codes, NDC (National Drug Code) numbers, and complete supplier information. A separate suppliers profile section provides information such as company address, telephone number, annual revenues, number of employees, names of top administrators, and product listings. In addition, the massive keyword index allows access to the volume by brand and generic name, drug class, therapeutic use, and some unique categories, such as date of FDA approval, pregnancy risk category, maintenance drugs, and lists of the 100 to 800 most prescribed drugs.

PROFESSIONAL SOURCES OF DRUG INFORMATION

Some of the best sources of drug information originate from professional societies. Their chief benefit lies in their authoritative evaluation. Professional groups, such as the American Society for Hospital Pharmacists and the American Medical Association (AMA), compile and evaluate information for their members. These tools are extremely valuable in the library setting.

10.14 *AHFS Drug Information*. Washington, DC, American Society of Hospital Pharmacists, 1959- .

10.15 *Drug Evaluations Annual*. Chicago, American Medical Association Department of Drugs and American Society for Clinical Pharmacology and Therapeutics. Annual. 1992- . Formerly: *AMA Drug Evaluations*.

10.16 *USP DI: United States Pharmacopeia Dispensing Information*. Rockville, MD, United States Pharmacopeial Convention, 1980- . Annual, bimonthly updates.

10.17 *Handbook of Nonprescription Drugs*. 9th ed. Washington, DC, American Pharmaceutical Association and National Professional Society of Pharmacists, 1991.

Formerly known as the *American Hospital Formulary Service Drug Information*, *AHFS Drug Information* is produced by the American Society of Hospital Pharmacists. It is designed to be a current collection of unbiased and evaluated monographs for pharmacists and other members of the medical community. *AHFS* is arranged by class of drug, for example, antineoplastic agents, cardiovascular drugs, hormones, and synthetic substitutes. Each section begins with a listing of the generic names found in that section. This listing can be helpful when spellings are doubtful. For example, a medical student interested in "decarbazine," an antineoplastic agent, would find the correct spelling, "dacarbazine," in consulting *AHFS*. Each monograph includes alternate name; chemical structural formula; descriptive sections on pharmacology, absorption, distribution, metabolism, and excretion; uses; cautions; dosage; and proprietary preparations that include the agent.

Investigational uses of approved drugs are included, as are some nonprescription agents such as vitamins. Many sections have an introductory statement about the class of drugs; for example, the section on radiopharmaceuticals has a general statement about the physics of radioactivity, radiation effects, and radiation protection. A classification number is assigned to each drug; and in the index, both generic and trade names refer to classification number. Supplements are issued several times a year. The evaluation process is excellent but tends to delay the speed with which new drugs are added. There are no bibliographies in the print source, but the electronic equivalent, Drug Info Fulltext, does provide bibliographic citations. Drug Info Fulltext includes *AHFS* as well as the more specialized *Handbook of Injectable Drugs* and is available through DIALOG and BRS.

Drug Evaluations Annual was formerly known as *AMA Drug Evaluations*, a title that was more suggestive of the therapeutic focus of this source. The work is a joint effort of the American Medical Association Department of Drugs and the American Society for Clinical Pharmacology and Therapeutics. It is intended to correlate current scientific findings on drugs and relate them to clinical practice decisions. *Drug Evaluations Annual* lists uses, routes of administration, and dosages, which may or may not be found in the package insert. The source attempts to describe all scientifically recognized uses of a given agent, regardless of the package insert. Again, information in this work is arranged by therapeutic class. Each section begins with general statements on the conditions requiring treatment and then gives individual evaluations of various drugs used in treatment, including dosage and preparations available. Two notable aspects are the evaluation of mixtures of drugs and the emphasis on the treatment of a condition or disease, including related material on diet. The index, by brand or generic name, disease, or symptom, is in the center of the volume.

The *USP DI: United States Pharmacopeia Dispensing Information* was introduced by the U.S. Pharmacopeia to provide prescribing and dispensing information not included in the official compendia (*see* 10.18), for example, precautions, side effects, and dosage. Volume 1 was written for the health care provider and volume 2 (*see* 10.34) was written in lay language to be used as an aid to patient consultation. A third volume, *Approved Drug Products and Legal Requirements,* contains the FDA's "Orange Book" (*Approved Drug Products with Therapeutic Equivalence Evaluations*) as well as selected federal laws and regulations useful to the pharmacist. This third volume can be used to see if a prescription or nonprescription drug has been approved by the FDA and the date in which each of its forms (liquid, tablet, etc.) was approved. The volume also provides therapeutic equivalence evaluations for approved generics, which may be available from a number of manufacturers. This information allows pharmacists to decide which generics can be safely substituted for others.

The *Handbook of Nonprescription Drugs,* published by the American Pharmaceutical Association and the National Professional Society of Pharmacists, deals only with over-the-counter or nonprescription products. Although the lay public assumes that no harm can come from the use of nonprescription drugs, in reality there are certain dangers. This book addresses those dangers. Each chapter deals with a therapeutic use—for example, laxative products, infant formula products, contact lens products, sunscreen products—in short, any product that may be purchased without prescription. The chapters describe the condition and the mechanism of action of available products. Often they include useful charts comparing the preparations. Before OTC product manufacturers were required to list all ingredients on the label, this source was useful for comparative purposes; for example, to determine which shampoos contain hexachlorophene. Although it is still useful for this purpose, it is perhaps most used now for its overview of nonprescription remedies.

OFFICIAL COMPENDIA

A pharmacopeia is an official book of legal pharmaceutical standards. Countries publish pharmacopeias to define the purity and standards of chemicals used in therapy. Often included are references to chemical tests and assay methods.

10.18 *The United States Pharmacopeia.* 22d rev. ed. *The National Formulary.* 17th ed. Rockville, MD, United States Pharmacopeial Convention, 1990.

The two official compendia recognized in the United States are *The U.S. Pharmacopeia (USP)* and *The National Formulary (NF).* These two publications have both been publishing official standards since 1820 and 1888, respectively, although under different sponsorship. After publication of the *National Formulary XIV,* the *NF* was acquired by the U.S. Pharmacopeial Convention; beginning in 1979, the two were published in one volume. The volume provides physical and chemical properties of a drug, including information on how to store, label, and analyze the substance.

The U.S. Pharmacopeia and *The National Formulary* contain much useful information, and pharmacopeias from other countries are actually little needed by most health sciences librarians in the United States unless users in a particular library require a heavy emphasis on pharmacy and the manufacture of drugs. The need to collect pharmacopeias from other countries is, in fact, often misinterpreted. Most drug questions relate to therapeutic use or to the general identification of a drug, rather than to standards of purity as given in these compendia. However, caution should be exercised in evaluating any title including the word "pharmacopeia." *Martindale: The Extra Pharmacopeia (see 10.9),* for example, is not really a pharmacopeia in the true sense of the word because it is not a listing of legal standards.

ADVERSE EFFECTS, TOXICOLOGY, POISONING

Some of the most commonly asked questions concern the untoward effects of drugs and chemicals: What are the adverse effects of indomethacin? What is the lethal dose of aspirin? Is it safe to drink alcohol if I'm taking Zantac? A number of previously described sources give some of this information, but other tools should also be considered.

10.19 Dukes, M.N.G. *Meyler's Side Effects of Drugs: An Encyclopedia of Adverse Reactions and Interaction.* 12th ed. Amsterdam, The Netherlands, Elsevier, 1992.

10.20 *Side Effects of Drugs Annual: A Worldwide Yearly Survey of New Data and Trends.* Amsterdam, The Netherlands, Excerpta Medica. Vol. 1- , 1977- .

10.21 Shepard, Thomas H. *Catalog of Teratogenic Agents.* 7th ed. Baltimore, MD, Johns Hopkins University Press, 1992.

10.22 Briggs, G. G.; Freeman, Roger K.; and Yaffe, Sumner J. *Drugs in Pregnancy and Lactation; A Reference Guide to Fetal and Neonatal Risk.* 3rd ed. Baltimore, MD, William & Wilkins, 1990.

10.23 *Registry of Toxic Effects of Chemical Substances.* Cincinnati, OH, National Institute for Occupational Safety and Health, 1978- . Microfiche, quarterly; hardcopy, annual.

10.24 Gosselin, Robert E., et al. *Clinical Toxicology of Commercial Products: Acute Poisoning.* 5th ed. Baltimore, MD, William & Wilkins, 1984.

10.25 Lewis, Richard J. *Sax's Dangerous Properties of Industrial Materials.* 8th ed. New York, Van Nostrand Reinhold, 1992.

Meyler's Side Effects of Drugs includes comprehensive review articles that summarize side effects of drugs reported in the international literature. The information is selective and is reviewed critically. Indexes provide access from trade names, generic names, and type of side effect. After publication of the eighth volume, *Side Effects of Drugs Annual* was introduced to review side effects literature published between editions on a cumulative basis. Librarians should be aware that both *Meyler's* and its update refer heavily to earlier editions so that none should be discarded. The electronic database, SEDBASE (DIALOG), contains the full text of the last twelve years of *Meyler's* and *Side Effects of Drugs Annual,* as well as Marler's *Pharmacological & Chemical Synonyms* (*see* 10.30).

Increasingly, there is concern about effects of drugs on the human reproductive organs, the fetus (teratology), and the breast-feeding infant. Dr. Shepard has been compiling information on teratogens for more than twenty years, gathering citations from researchers all over the world. The *Catalog of Teratogenic Agents* covers fetal exposure to more than 2,000 drugs, chemicals, and physical agents. Electronically, it joins the Teratogen Information System (TERIS) in Micromedex's CCIS (*see* 10.40) as valuable tools to research the field.

As its name implies, *Drugs in Pregnancy and Lactation* includes not only information on possible harm to the fetus from drugs taken during pregnancy but difficulties encountered if a breast-feeding mother uses medication. Drugs are listed alphabetically under generic name (the index supplies cross-references from trade names). Each entry lists drug class, a coded fetal risk factor, and summaries of current knowledge on dangers to the fetus and breast-fed infant. Extensive bibliographies follow the entries.

Registry of Toxic Effects of Chemical Substances (RTECS) is prepared by the National Institute for Occupational Safety and Health (NIOSH) to identify all known toxic substances in our environment and to codify known toxic doses. It is arranged by chemical substance. The following information is included when available: CAS registry number, molecular weight and formula, toxic data, and U.S. and NIOSH documents citing standards for handling the substance. The toxic dose data include dose, route of administration or exposure, kind of effect, and published reference. This source is also available electronically on DIALOG and through the National Library of Medicine as part of TOXNET.

Clinical Toxicology of Commercial Products is specifically designed to provide toxicity and hazard information for chemicals contained in products used in the home and commercial setting. For example, it gives information on oven cleaners, hair spray, and artificial snow used to spray Christmas trees. The wide variety of product information includes sections on ingredients, trade names, and representative formulas. In addition, a special section on first aid and emergency care is provided, as are descriptions of therapeutic measures for selected classes of ingredients. Because this title is now dated, libraries that have Micromedex's POISINDEX (*see* 10.40) might prefer to consult that source.

Dangerous Properties of Industrial Materials rates various industrial chemicals, giving the chemical name, synonyms, molecular formula, and hazard analysis (toxicity, radiation hazards, and fire hazards). For example, vinyl chloride, a chemical frequently used in processing industries, is listed with a high hazard rating for exposure through inhalation. Countermeasures are listed; e.g., adequate ventilation is necessary when working with vinyl chloride. Also included are recommendations for storage, handling, and shipping.

This discussion of sources on poisoning would not be complete without a brief mention of poison control centers. The first poison control center was opened in 1953; since then, additional centers have been established. The National Clearinghouse for Poison Control Centers collects information on poisons and disseminates it throughout the country. The services of these centers are available to all physicians and, frequently, to the public; their aim is to provide prompt information on poisoning and its treatment. Standard reference works such as the *PDR* often include listings of poison control centers. However, librarians making referrals should be aware that the size and quality of the centers vary widely.

DRUG INTERACTIONS

An increasingly important area of drug information concerns the literature of drug interactions. It is becoming more evident that administering a drug coincidentally with another drug or chemical can affect the pharma-cological action. For example, procarbazine should not be taken with cheese or wine. Some drugs may effectively lose therapeutic potential if taken with another drug; others may have their bioavailability increased to toxic levels. Clearly, these interrelationships must be better understood and codified. The sources listed here are but examples of the types of publications addressing this need. Because there may be considerable variance both in coverage and evaluation, especially of more minor reactions, ideally more than one source should be consulted.

10.26 *Drug Interaction Facts.* St. Louis, MO, Lippincott. Loose-leaf. 1983-.
10.27 Zucchero, Frederic J.; Shinn, A.F.; and Hogan, Mark J., eds. *Evaluations of Drug Interactions.* 4th ed. New York, Macmillan. Loose-leaf. 1988- .
10.28 Hansten, Philip D. and Horn, J.R. *Drug Interactions: Clinical Significance of Drug-Drug Interactions and Drug Effects on Clinical Laboratory Results.* 6th ed. Philadelphia, Lea & Febiger, 1989. Loose-leaf.
10.29 *PDR Guide to Drug Interactions, Side Effects, Indications; keyed to PDR.* Montvale, NJ, Medical Economics. 1993- .

Drug Interaction Facts is probably the simplest to use of these sources. Produced by the Mediphor Group, it is arranged alphabetically by principal drug affected. It includes only the most important interactions, but for those it gives concise information on the significance and rapidity of the interaction, its severity, how well documented the interaction is, the mechanism of action, and suggested management. There is also a brief discussion of the interaction and references are included. The index is arranged by generic name but frequently provides cross-references from major trade names. Clinically substantiated interactions are indicated by bold type. *Drug Interaction Facts* is also available in electronic format as Interactive Drug Interactions from MEDISPAN, a section of Micromedex's CCIS (*see* 10.40).

Evaluations of Drug Interactions (EDI) was developed by the American Pharmaceutical Association. The book is arranged in chapters by drug category (e.g., antidepressant drug interactions). The first drug listed is altered by the second. Each entry includes a summary of the reaction, other related drugs for which the same reaction could be expected, mechanism of action, recommendations for management, and appropriate references. The severity of the reaction is coded at the end of the monograph, and the code appears in the index next to the major drugs discussed in the interaction (but not for the related drugs mentioned in the discussion). Like *Drug Interaction Facts,* the index provides cross-references from the more well-known trade names. A helpful appendix lists drugs by pharmacologic action (e.g., antihistamines). A summarized version of *EDI* is available on floppy disk from the publisher as MEDICOM MICRO. The software refers users to the print edition for more complete information.

Hansten's *Drug Interactions* is highly regarded by pharmacists but may be more difficult for the librarian to use because reactions are arranged and often indexed by class. For instance, users looking for an interaction between Pargyline and Anafranil (clomipramine) would find the needed information in a section discussing monoamine oxidase inhibitors with tricyclic antidepressants. However, before consulting *Drug Interactions*, the user would have to know that Pargyline is a monoamine oxidase inhibitor and Anafranil is a tricyclic antidepressant. For knowledgeable users, Hansten's *Drug Interactions* provides an overview of the mechanism, clinical significance, and management of the interaction. The reference list is extensive.

PDR Guide to Drug Interactions, Side Effects, Indications; keyed to PDR can be useful in identifying interactions, especially minor interactions, that are included in the *PDR* series. This source does not stand alone but refers to the page in the *PDR* set (*PDR, PDR for Nonprescription Drugs, PDR for Ophthalmic Drugs*) where more complete information may be found. Entry is by food-drug interaction, by drug-drug interaction, or by side effect (*see* 10.11 for a more complete description of the *PDR* series).

FOREIGN DRUGS

Questions about foreign drugs often are particularly vexing. For example, spelling may vary in different languages. Users often have insufficient information, and the librarian begins a search looking for the proverbial needle in the haystack. Whenever possible, the requester should be queried for further information: Do you have the exact spelling of the drug name? Do you know the country of origin? For what purpose is the drug used? Do you know the manufacturer?

Several sources described earlier are very useful for foreign drug names. *Martindale: The Extra Pharmacopoeia* is extremely valuable for its wide coverage of European drugs and extensive indexing under trade names. *The Merck Index* is useful because of its broad international coverage and its inclusion of many chemical, generic, and even trade names. *Unlisted Drugs* should also be consulted and is particularly useful because it covers many years through the *Unlisted Drug Index Guide*.

Three other sources are particularly helpful for foreign drug identification.

10.30 Marler, E. E. J. *Pharmacological and Chemical Synonyms: A Collection of Drugs, Pesticides, and Other Compounds Drawn from the Literature of the World.* 9th ed. New York, Elsevier, 1990.

10.31 *International Drug Directory 1992/93.* Zurich, Switzerland, Societe Suisse de Pharmacie, 1992. Formerly: *Index Nominum* (French).

10.32 Schlesser, Jerry L., ed. *Drugs Available Abroad: A Guide to Therapeutic Drugs Available and Approved Outside the U.S.* Detroit, Gale, 1990.

Marler's *Pharmacological and Chemical Synonyms* is essentially an alphabetical list. It contains more than 10,000 drugs and chemicals as well as 50,000 international synonyms, including research codes and trade names. *International Drug Directory* (formerly in French and known as *Index Nominum*) goes a bit further. All listings are under the World Health Organization's International Nonproprietary Name with the following information: chemical name, molecular and structural formula, Chemical Abstract Service registry numbers, therapeutic class, generic names, official names, and trade names.

Drugs Available Abroad is limited in scope to drugs not approved in the United States—either because the drugs have not yet completed the lengthy testing procedure required by the FDA or because the manufacturers have chosen not to apply for FDA approval because of the time and expense involved. Foreign here means Europe, the Caribbean, Central America, Mexico, Australia, Canada, and South Africa. The concise descriptions include generic and trade names, dosage information, contraindications, adverse effects, country where available, release date, and information on the drug's current status in the FDA approval process. An especially valuable feature is the identification of U. S. approved drugs that may serve as therapeutic equivalents. The preface includes a description of procedures for exporting or importing unapproved drugs. There are indexes by drug name, clinical indication, manufacturer, and country in use. Although far from complete, this source is easy to understand and use.

Librarians needing more extensive coverage may want to consider indexes focusing on drugs available in a particular country, such as *Compendium of Pharmaceuticals* (Canada) or *Diccionario de Especialidades Farmaceuticas* (Mexico). In addition, online services often can be used advantageously for foreign drug names. These names may appear in the title or in the abstract. In the case of the Excerpta Medica system, there is a field specifically designated for trade names. With online systems, it is possible to "neighbor" a term to see if there are variant spellings. The cross-file finding databases (Product Name Finder or DIALINDEX on DIALOG and CROS on BRS) may also prove helpful in locating databases that mention the drug.

DRUG INFORMATION FOR PATIENTS AND THE PUBLIC

As indicated previously, the consumer movement in the United States has greatly increased the public's "desire to know." Health sciences librarians are frequently asked drug information questions by the general public and, accordingly, each library must decide its own policy for responding to these questions. Most materials are very technical, and the general writing style usually does not lend itself to easy interpretation. The librarian should always exercise discretion and encourage requesters to consult with a health care practitioner to interpret and evaluate their questions.

10.33 *Medication Teaching Manual.* 5th ed. Washington, DC, American Society of Hospital Pharmacists, 1991.

10.34 *USP DI v. 2 Advice For the Patient; Drug Information in Lay Language.* 13th ed. Rockville, MD, U. S. Pharmacopeial Convention, 1993.

10.35 Long, James W. *Essential Guide to Prescription Drugs, 1993.* New York, HarperPerennial, 1993.

10.36 Griffith, H. Winter. *Complete Guide to Prescription & Non-prescription Drugs.* New York, Body Press/Perigee, 1992.

Patient noncompliance with drug therapy has been recognized for a long time. Often patients lack an understanding of what they have been prescribed to take and why. They are frequently confused and concerned about side effects that might occur. Consequently, there have been a number of attempts to develop educational materials for patients. Two notable efforts include the *USP DI (see* 10.16) volume entitled *Advice for the Patient* and the American Society of Hospital Pharmacists' *Medication Teaching Manual.* These publications, reviewed by drug experts, are designed to answer patient questions. The *USP DI* volume is especially useful; it is clearly written and provides information on precautions, proper use and storage of medication, and the frequency of side effects (including whether they are significant enough to warrant consulting a physician). Drugs are indexed by generic and trade name. Although not complete, a photographic section does group drugs alphabetically by generic name. Users can consult this section to verify that the blue 150 mg amitriptyline they formerly took as Elavil should be the same as the green Geneva tablet marked GG 450. *USP DI Advice for the Patient* is also sold by Consumer Reports Books under the title *The Complete Drug Reference.* This title was rated the number-one drug information book for consumers in a recent *US News & World Report* survey. In addition, a condensed version of this work is available under the title *About Your Medicines.*

Commercial sources such as *Essential Guide to Prescription Drugs* are also helpful. Although not as complete as *USP DI Advice for the Patient* (which includes more prescription drugs as well as some nonprescription medications), Long's volume is very clear. It lists drugs individually under generic name (*USP DI* frequently discusses similar drugs by class group although the index provides access by drug name). In addition, Long provides some unique features (e.g., effects of the drug on sexual function, possible interactions with lab tests) which are very useful. An additional section entitled "Essential Guide to Prescription Drugs" gives overviews on common diseases, including drugs used to treat them.

Another excellent source is H. Winter Griffith's *Complete Guide to Prescription and Non-Prescription Drugs*. Dr. Griffith is widely known for his work in patient education. The work is updated annually and provides basic information on both prescription and nonprescription medications, including combination drugs.

In addition, many other drug information titles are aimed at the consumer. The *Consumer Health Information Source Book* by Alan Rees and Catherine Hoffman (3d ed. Phoenix, AZ: Oryx Press, 1990) provides an annotated list of possibilities although, of course, it does not include newer offerings such as the *PDR Family Guide to Prescription Drugs* (Montvale, NJ: Medical Economics, 1993).

INDEXING AND ABSTRACTING SERVICES AND ELECTRONIC DATABASES

Indexing and abstracting services and online databases are described in Chapters 4 and 5. However, some indexing and abstracting services that are specific to drug information should be noted.

The National Library of Medicine's *MeSH (Medical Subject Headings)* (*see* Chapters 4 and 5) has shown a dramatic increase in its inclusion of drug names since its inception. Earliest editions relied heavily on classes of chemical compounds. Each year, however, many specific drug names have been added to Section D, "Chemicals and Drugs." Today, approximately 40% of total MeSH descriptors belong in Section D.

MeSH entries for drugs are generic names. In a few cases, when the trade name is very common, there is a cross-reference from the trade name to the generic MeSH term. Therefore, for the user of *Index Medicus*, tools such as the *American Drug Index* or *USAN and the USP Dictionary of Drug Names* may often be needed to convert a trade name to a generic name. Sometimes the drug name may be a minor descriptor; to find information in the printed *Index Medicus*, it will be necessary to use a broader name representing a class of drugs. Because drug names have been added so frequently to *MeSH*, the user must pay special attention to entry dates for MeSH terms.

Often it is useful to determine when a drug became an official USAN (or INN, if it is a foreign drug). This will give an indication of a realistic time period for a search. For example, nizatidine, an antiulcerative agent, became a USAN in 1983, a provisional MeSH descriptor in 1985, and a full descriptor in 1992. To search *Index Medicus* prior to 1992, one would look under the heading "THIAZOLES," because the term nizatadine is only a provisional heading. Because other thiazoles are indexed in the same place, it would be necessary to scan for article titles that mention nizatidine or its trade name, Axid. For a MEDLINE search, "NIZATIDINE" will suffice back through 1985; but for previous years, especially before 1983, when the USAN was approved, the search would have to include nizatidine as a textword, the trade name, other synonyms, and research code names. For the years before a drug is officially named, *Biological Abstracts* (*see* Chapter 4) and *Chemical Abstracts* (*see* Chapter 4) or their electronic counterparts may be more useful sources.

In other cases, information may be needed about the drug therapy of a specific disease or chemicals causing a disease. In those cases, the subheadings "drug therapy" and "chemically induced" are especially useful in searching both *Index Medicus* and MEDLINE. The librarian should be familiar with all the subheadings applicable to Section D of *MeSH*.

TOXLINE (*see* 5.2), a prime tool to locate toxicology information, also includes a variety of nontoxicologic information. Its inclusion of the pharmacodynamics section of *Biological Abstracts* and *International Pharmaceutical Abstracts* makes it a good source of general drug information.

Other NLM databases of interest to drug specialists include CHEMLINE (*see* 5.3), CHEMID (*see* 5.4), RTECS (*see* 5.20), and CANCERLIT (*see* 5.6). CHEMLINE or CHEMID can be used quite effectively when constructing search terms for natural language databases, including TOXLINE. The online version of RTECS (Registry of Toxic Effects of Chemical Substances) is much easier to use than the printed version and is more timely. CANCERLIT, which includes records from NLM and the International Cancer Research Data Bank (ICRDB) of the National Cancer Institute, may be a good place to look for information on investigational drugs used in treating neoplasms. Another database developed by the ICRDB, PDQ (Physician's Data Query), can provide information on standard cancer drug protocols and lists clinical trials using that drug.

Chemical Abstracts (*see* 4.15) is also a useful source of information. Many of the biochemistry sections (e.g., pharmacodynamics, hormone pharmacology, toxicology, biochemical interactions) include drug information material. In the macromolecular chemistry sections, there are two of interest: pharmaceuticals and pharmaceutical analysis. Many of the sections relating to industrial chemistry include references to occupational hazards. When searching *Chemical Abstracts* for a particular drug, the *Index Guide* should be consulted to find the correct index term. Specific chemicals are included in the chemical substance index. Ribavirin, for example, is indexed under 1H-1, 2, 4-triazole-3-carboxamide, -1-B-D-ribofuranosyl-. Classes of chemicals and other concepts, such as "antibiotics" and "brain neoplasms," are indexed in the general subject index. Because of its great breadth, *Chemical Abstracts* is often used to locate citations not indexed elsewhere. Patents describing the manufacture of a specific drug fall into this category. Although the emphasis is not primarily on clinical medicine, extensive research material is included and there is substantial coverage of drugs in research. When using *Chemical Abstracts* as an electronic database, the CAS registry number for the compound may provide one of the most efficient ways of searching a drug with multiple names.

> 10.37 *Excerpta Medica. Drug Literature Index.* Section 37. Amsterdam, The Netherlands, Excerpta Medica, 1980- . (Published as *Drug Literature Index* since 1969).
> 10.38 *International Pharmaceutical Abstracts: Key to the World's Literature of Pharmacy.* Washington, DC, American Society of Hospital Pharmacists. Vol. 1- , 1964- . Semimonthly.
> 10.39 *Inpharma: Weekly Reports from the Current International Drug Literature.* Auckland, New Zealand, ADIS Press. No. 1- , 1975- .

Many of the Excerpta Medica abstracting services include pharmacologic information. The Excerpta Medica Foundation has gathered all drug-related articles in Section 37, *Drug Literature Index*, which has special indexes for classification codes, pharmaceutical or generic names, trade names, new drugs, and author names. In parallel manner, the online version of Excerpta Medica, EMBASE (*see* 5.26), is an excellent source for drug information. EMBASE Drug Information, a new database available through BRS, is a subset of the larger EMBASE and contains documents from the *Pharmacology, Drug Literature Index*, and *Adverse Reactions Titles* sections. The advantages EMBASE offers over MEDLINE include more international coverage; frequently, more specific headings (e.g., separate headings for dosage and administration); and more detailed drug indexing (EMBASE indexes the trade names and routes of drug administration for all articles in which these aspects are mentioned). On the other hand, MEDLINE is considerably less costly to search and the journals indexed are frequently easier to obtain.

The semimonthly *International Pharmaceutical Abstracts (IPA)* covers many areas of interest to pharmacists and drug information specialists, including pharmaceutical technology, the practice of pharmacy, investigational drugs, drug testing and analysis, drug stability, and pharmaceutical chemistry. Cumulative indexes are published every six months, and three-year cumulative indexes were published from 1978-1986. Journal coverage includes many basic medical journals as well as sources not included in

Index Medicus. Examples of the latter include *American Druggist, Drugs &
Society,* and *Pharmaceutical Manufacturing. IPA* is useful for finding information on topics such as drug information services, drug sales, drug preparation, and chemical data (for example, articles discussing the half-life or
stability of a drug). *International Pharmaceutical Abstracts* can also be
searched electronically and is available in CD-ROM format.

  Inpharma: Weekly Reports from the Current International Drug Literature has
been published since 1975 by ADIS Press. The editors of this newsletter
select and summarize very recent articles on drugs in clinical use; its chief
value is as a current tool for alerting pharmacists and others involved in
drug therapy. Most issues include a section on drugs newly introduced in
various countries of the world and summary listings of articles on selected
topics. There are quarterly, six-month, and annual indexes to *Inpharma* by
generic name, disease state, and general terms, such as hepatotoxicity and
pregnancy. New product introductions are cumulated and drug interactions are combined under one heading. *Inpharma* appears full text (with the
publication *Reactions,* which focuses on adverse drug reactions) on BRS as
ADIS Drug News.

  In addition to the databases already mentioned, there are a number of
more specialized online services of interest to pharmaceutical searchers.
These are detailed in Table 10-2. Frequently, questions will deal with finding
information on the approval status of a new drug or locating sales or
personnel information for a particular pharmaceutical company. A number
of databases, including Diogenes, F-D-C Reports, Health News Daily,
Pharmaceutical and Healthcare Industry News (PHIND), and Pharmaceu-
tical News Index, target pharmaceutical news of this nature. In addition to
IPA, bibliographic databases specific to pharmacy include IDIS (Iowa Drug
Information Service), Pharmaceutical Literature Documentation
(RINGDOC), and ADIS Alerts. The handbooks available full-text online
include Beilstein Online, Consumer Drug Information (*Consumer Drug
Digest*), Drug Information Fulltext (*Handbook on Injectable Drugs, AHFS
Drug Information*), Martindale Online, Merck Index, Registry of Toxic Effects
of Chemical Substances, and SEDBASE (*Meyler's Side Effects of Drugs; Side
Effects of Drugs Annual;* Marler's *Pharmacological & Chemical Synonyms*).
Pharmacontacts provides directory information on pharmaceutical companies and organizations. Pharmaprojects is unique in listing the worldwide
status of a drug (Phase I testing, approved, etc.) and is very useful for its
thorough inclusion of drug synonyms. Unfortunately, there are significant
viewing charges for users who do not subscribe to the print version of this
product.

  Many electronic databases are now also available as CD-ROM products.
Among those especially useful to researchers in the field of drugs are
MEDLINE (many versions); Biological Abstracts; CHEM-BANK (hazard-

Table 10-2. Online Resources for Drug Information

FILE	PRINT EQUIVALENT	EMPHASIS
ADIS Alerts Online (BRS)	None	Summaries of drug literature
ADIS Drug News (BRS)	*InPharma* and *Reactions*	New drugs
Aidsdrugs (MEDLARS)	None	Investigational AIDS drugs
Beilstein Online (DLG)	*Beilstein's Handbuch der Organischen Chemie*	Chemical properties
Consumer Drug Information (DLG)	*Consumer Drug Digest*	Information in laymen's language
De Haen's Drug Data (Several)	None	Journal & report literature
Derwent Ringdoc (DLG)	None	Journal literature on pharmaceutics
Diogenes (Several)	None—indexes unpublished FDA documents plus selected full-text newsletters	Full-text information on drugs
Drug Information Fulltext (Several)	*Handbook on Injectable Drugs; AHFS Drug Information; FDA Drug Bulletin*	Full-text articles
F-D-C Reports (DLG)	Full-text of FDC newsletters ("Pink sheet," "Gray sheet," "Rose sheet," *FDA Drug & Device Product Approvals*)	FDA regulatory information, news
Health News Daily (Several)	Same	Pharmaceutical industry news; political emphasis
International Pharmaceutical Abstracts (IPA) (Several)	Same	All aspects of pharmacy
Iowa Drug Information Service (IDIS) (BRS)	Same	Journal articles on drugs
Martindale Online (DLG)	*Martindale: The Extra Pharmacopoeia*	Full-text drug monographs

Table 10-2. Online Resources for Drug Information (continued)

FILE	PRINT EQUIVALENT	EMPHASIS
Pharmaceutical & Healthcare Industry News (PHIND) (Several)	Includes full-text *SCRIP, CLINICA* newsletters	Pharmaceutical industry news
Pharmaceutical News Index (PNI) (Several)	Full-text of several newsletters	Pharmaceutical industry news
Pharmacontacts (BRS)	None	Directory
Pharmaprojects (Several)	Same	Status of drug; drug synonyms worldwide
SEDBASE (Several)	*Meyler's Side Effects of Drugs; Side Effects of Drugs Annual;* Marler's *Pharmacological & Chemical Synonyms*	Adverse effects of drugs
21 CFR Online (BRS)	*Code of Federal Regulations*	Federal regulations on drugs

ous substances); Drug Information Source Database (includes *Drug Information Fulltext, AHFS Drug Information, Handbook on Injectable Drugs, International Pharmaceutical Abstracts*); Drugs and Pharmacology (citations and abstracts on drugs and pharmacology from 3,500 biomedical journals, 1980- .); Excerpta Medica CD: Drugs and Pharmacology; International Pharmaceutical Abstracts; and Physicians Desk Reference on CD-ROM.

10.40 *Computerized Clinical Information System (CCIS)*. Denver, CO, Micromedex. Quarterly.

Another expensive but very useful source is the CD-ROM product, Computerized Clinical Information System (CCIS) from Micromedex. CCIS is also available for use on a mainframe and some sections are searchable through MEDIS. The full set includes more than 20 subfiles which can also be purchased in various combinations. Many sections are composed of long monographs providing a full-text overview of current knowledge on a drug or a condition seen in an emergency room setting. A system of menus guides the user to the correct section of the monograph. Lengthy bibliographies at the end of each monograph are selective rather than exhaustive. Most subfiles offer multiple methods of access, including generic and trade names, foreign drug names, symptoms caused or treated by the drug, and even tablet imprint. The sections of most interest to drug information professionals include

POISINDEX (information on treating drug or chemical substance overdose/ingestion).

IDENTIDEX (identifying a drug through the imprint on the tablet or capsule).

DRUGDEX System-Drug Evaluation Monographs (overview of a drug).

DRUGDEX System-Drug Consults (short articles on specific topics, e.g., should scopalomine patches for seasickness be cut in half).

Martindale: The Extra Pharmacopeia (electronic version of *Martindale* [*see* 10.9]).

Material Safety Data Sheets (physical and health hazards of drugs and chemicals, especially dangers involved in handling the substance).

Interactive Drug Interactions from MEDISPAN (electronic version of *Drug Interaction Facts* [*see* 10.26] which allows up to fifteen drugs to be checked simultaneously in all permutations).

Aftercare Instructions (information for the consumer, electronic version of *USP DI v. 2 Advice for the Patient* [*see* 10.34]; also available in low literacy and Spanish versions).

REPRORISK—TERIS (short reviews on the effects of drugs and chemicals on the fetus); and

REPRORISK—Shepard's *Catalog of Teratogenic Agents* (electronic version of well-known print source, *see* 10.21).

DRUG INFORMATION SERVICES

As pharmacists' roles have expanded from the dispensing of medications to more active participation in patient care, more hospitals are forming drug information services that provide specialized information about drugs to the medical and nursing staffs. Pharmacists working in the drug information service will answer detailed questions arising during patient care, will provide a continuing educational medium by reviewing publications on drugs, and will analyze literature to arrive at a conclusion when conflicting information exists. They may extend their services to other health professionals in the community or even to the general public.

These drug information services often use reference sources that only very specialized libraries might carry. One is Micromedex's CCIS (10.40) and another is the Iowa Drug Information Service, which is available with either a manual or a computer index to access a full-text microfiche library.

Librarians should be aware of local drug information services in nearby hospitals. Although the recent trend among drug information services to charge for their work may complicate the relationship, both librarians and drug information staff should work together to satisfy users' needs.

READINGS

Abate MA, Jacknowitz AI, Shumway JM. Information sources utilized by private practice and university physicians. Drug Inf J 1989;23:309-19.

Beaird SL, Coley RM, Crea KA. Current status of drug information centers. Amer J Hosp Pharm 1992;19(1):103-6.

Findlay S. Best books. US News World Rep 1991;110(19):80-2.

Murdoch LL. Foreign drug identification. DICP 1989;23:501-6.

Urdang G. The development of pharmacopoeias. Bull WHO 1951;4:577-603.

CHAPTER 11

Audiovisual, Microcomputer, and Multimedia Reference Sources

Diane P. Futrelle and James A. Curtis

Quality audiovisual, microcomputer, and multimedia information services can be provided with access to a combination of current print sources, external online search services, electronic information networks, and human resource networks of biomedical communication and educational technology professionals. Reference sources for audiovisual, microcomputer, and multimedia software are published in print and electronic formats. Each format, ranging from ephemeral brochures to online databases, serves a valuable purpose in supporting reference and collection development services.

It is important to use frequently updated and current reference sources because the nature of most hardware and software questions pertain to new technology and recently produced materials. Changes in educational technology, coupled with the rapid evolution of the subject matter, require current sources to identify educational materials. As numerous producers of educational materials and reference tools go in and out of business, so do the publishers of reference guides, databases, and review publications. Therefore, the scope of this chapter includes only sources published or updated within the last five years.

Reference sources that exclusively describe one format of information, such as audiovisual or microcomputer software, are becoming progressively rare. Online databases more frequently index both print and nonprint materials. Audiovisual databases are now more likely to include microcomputer and multimedia titles. Film and media festivals are becoming inclusive of all media formats. Software no longer refers to audiovisuals but is a generic term for information stored in a magnetic, electronic, or digital form. It is becoming more prevalent that the same title or body of information will be distributed in various formats and platforms. Although every attempt was made to group the reference sources described in this chapter into one of three broad categories—audiovisual, microcomputer, or multimedia—the boundaries of these divisions are melding and in many cases overlap.

CHARACTERISTICS

Audiovisual, Microcomputer, and Multimedia Collections

Over the past decade, nonprint collections in health sciences libraries have evolved from audiovisual collections to learning resources collections. The types of materials generally collected by media services, audiovisual services, and learning resources centers now include microcomputer software, courseware, and multimedia in addition to traditional audiovisual formats. Libraries often support the use of general purpose microcomputer software—such as word processing, bibliographic formatting, database management, graphic, statistical, and spreadsheet—and consider these tools to be part of the larger information management picture. The ideal microcomputer learning center or lab integrates the use of courseware and multimedia with other electronic information resources, creating a scholar's or physician's workstation concept.

Nonprint collections are generally characterized as "working collections." They are curriculum-based and, as such, are updated to support or supplement educational programs within the institution. Most health sciences media collections never become archival, because very few libraries can justify the expense of retaining audiovisual and courseware materials unrelated to an ongoing educational program or that have been replaced by updated versions. In a working collection there is heavy reliance on recent material, due to continuous changes in curricular content resulting from new knowledge or through changes in educational goals and faculty interests. Therefore, this chapter will focus on current reference sources describing materials in print or available to rent or borrow. Directories and print guides that are no longer updated that contain materials that are unavailable to purchase, out-of-date, or obsolete were excluded from this review.

Audiovisual, Microcomputer, and Multimedia Reference Requests

There are some characteristics that all media reference questions have in common and others that are particular to the desired format. Questions pertaining to the bibliographic and physical description, audience level, production dates, procurement source, and cost apply to all information requests about nonprint materials. Typical questions pertaining to audiovisual materials might include

A professor is looking for a set of slides on mouth neoplasms or oral cancer to accompany a lecture within two weeks for resident oncologists.

A student is going on a weeklong trip and would like to review any internal medicine topics for the board review. What appropriate audiocassette programs are available?

A physician is looking for some audiovisual programs that are eligible for continuing medical education (CME) and produced within the last two years within the medical specialty of cardiology.

A nurse would like to know the title, producer, and cost of a 1/2-inch videocassette program on the most current CPR procedure.

A faculty member would like to know what audiovisual, microcomputer, or multimedia programs on normal and abnormal heart sounds are available and which can be studied independently by students.

A hospital library is looking for a loan source for a video about the life and research of Elizabeth Kubler-Ross.

As part of the reference interview, the staff should collect the information on an information request form (Figure 11-1) before a search is conducted. If the reference request pertains to a subject search for nonprint materials, then all of the questions should be asked of the user. The audiovisual format is important not only for content and purpose, but also for the situation in which the program will be used. The intended audience level should be specified in order to identify the appropriate level of instruction. Broad audience levels could include higher education, undergraduate education, continuing education, in-service, staff development, patient education, health professional, and specific health sciences disciplines and medical specialties.

Characteristics Particular to Microcomputer and Multimedia Reference Requests

Responses to a second set of questions must be collected before a search for microcomputer and multimedia information can be conducted. These characteristics generally pertain to the hardware requirements and the computing environment in which the program will be installed and accessed. Because these questions are specific to electronic formats and do not apply to audiovisuals, they should be collected on the reverse side of the information request form or on a separate form. Typical questions pertaining to microcomputer and multimedia programs might include

Figure 11-1. Sample Information Request Form

(Includes characteristics common to all audiovisual, microcomputer, and multimedia reference questions)

Bibliographic and Physical Description:
Title
Broad subject
MeSH terms
Keywords
Producer/distributor
Format
Size
Length or run time
Color or black & white

Level:
Intended audience
Continuing education credit
Self-instructional or group

Dates:
Show date
Date not needed after
Production year range
Loan period

Procurement Source and Costs:
Preview or purchase
Borrow or rent
Access
Fee or free
Maximum fee

The Nutrition Department would like to know what diet analysis computer programs have recently been produced that run on a DOS platform in a Novell network environment.

A nursing faculty would like to identify some computer-based clinical simulations on the subject of nursing care of the elderly patient. She would like a program that can summarize and print the student and class responses.

The Office of Educational Development would like to know what interactive videodisc (IVD) programs have been developed that are compatible with the generic videodisc program "Slice of Life" running on a Macintosh platform.

A physician is looking for a computer assisted program on preventive methods in coronary heart disease that is eligible for continuing medical education credit.

A biostatistics student would like to know which statistical programs can be used to calculate and plot a regression analysis using a stand-alone IBM Model 30 computer without a hard disk.

What is the most recent version of Quick Medical Reference (QMR), and what is the price for a site license?

Requests to preview or purchase microcomputer and multimedia software should be treated a little differently than requests about software use in the library. In addition to the information collected for all nonprint reference questions previously mentioned, the library staff should also inquire as to how these programs will be used and in which computing environment. License agreements usually restrict the use of microcomputer software to one workstation, one computer lab, or a specific number of workstations on a network. Therefore, the answers to the following questions should be collected prior to conducting a search for educational software.

Computer platform
System requirements
Disk size
Disk density
Memory requirements
Networkable
Multiuser
Site license
Copy protection
Public domain or shareware
Peripheral requirements
Manual or user guide
Installation instructions

BIBLIOGRAPHIC CONTROL OF NONPRINT MATERIALS

The lack of bibliographic control for audiovisual, microcomputer, and multimedia materials hinders the identification of relevant software. There is no national trade bibliography equivalent to *Books in Print* for media. While audiovisual and microcomputer software should be treated like other library materials and cataloged according to standard AACR2 rules, no single source, including the AVLINE database, provides comprehensive coverage.

In response to the users' need to know what software is available in the library, specialized lists and bibliographies are very useful tools. Software bibliographies and mediographies are especially valuable in pulling together audiovisual and microcomputer programs available on frequently requested broad subject areas such as pregnancy and birth, death and dying, gerontology and aging, communications and management, nutrition, and wellness. Bibliographies also serve the purpose of identifying the numerous subject headings that may be associated with a broad subject or area of specialization. Lists created with database management software allow for greater flexibility in generating subsets such as all Macintosh, all CAI (Computer Assisted Instruction), or all interactive videodisc [1]. Indexes or arrangements by title, format, serial number, or subject can be easily created with database management software.

AUDIOVISUAL REFERENCE SOURCES

Primary Sources

Information about available audiovisual and microcomputer software appears first in the brochures or catalogs of the producers or distributors of health sciences media. Presently there are more than 1,000 producers and distributors of health sciences audiovisual materials. These brochures and catalogs form the primary, and sometimes the only, audiovisual reference sources. Catalogs are important because reference tools based upon them may provide insufficient information on which to make a judgment regarding acquisition. Libraries that support the curriculum and continuing education needs of several health sciences schools or medical disciplines will need to collect and index the full spectrum of producer catalogs. Program indexes, directories, and online databases do not replace a collection of producer and distributor catalogs. Lack of specific information in most audiovisual indexes, especially ordering information, reinforces the need to provide a collection of current producer brochures. Names and addresses of current audiovisual and microcomputer producers and distributors are best identified from the producer or distributor indexes of the primary references sources described in the following paragraphs.

Online Audiovisual Databases

11.1 *AVLINE (AudioVisuals onLINE)*. Bethesda, MD, National Library of Medicine, 1975- .

11.2 *A-V Online*. Albuquerque, NM, National Information Center for Educational Media, Access Innovations, 1964- .

The National Library of Medicine's (NLM) AVLINE database and the publications derived from it provide the best source of bibliographic and procurement information to more than 19,000 audiovisual and microcomputer software programs in all health sciences discipline areas. The National Library of Medicine is responsible for identifying, acquiring, and supplying bibliographic descriptions for the citations to health sciences audiovisual materials and, now, microcomputer software in the AVLINE database, which is part of the extensive MEDLARS network. There were four computer-produced publications derived from the AVLINE database, of which only the first is now updated and available in print.

National Library of Medicine Audiovisuals Catalog: 1977- .
National Library of Medicine AVLINE Catalog: 1975-76.
National Medical Audiovisual Center Catalog: Films for the Health Sciences: 1981.
Health Sciences Audiovisuals: microfiche only, ceased publication December 1988.

A-V Online is produced by the National Information Center for Educational Media (NICEM) and distributed in an online database, CD-ROM, and microfiche format by separate vendors. DIALOG offers access to the online version as file number 46, indexing more than 350,000 titles. NICEM acquires and encodes information on nonprint media covering all levels of education and instruction, beginning with preschool and ranging to postgraduate level materials, in all academic areas. Examples of extensively covered subject areas of particular interest to the health sciences are health and safety education; science; psychology; and athletics, physical education, and fitness. Citations include annotations and subject descriptors, audience level, and name and address of commercial source. Although NICEM has compiled the world's largest online index of information on audiovisual materials, it is not a comprehensive resource for the health sciences. It fails to cover numerous health sciences audiovisual producers and distributors geared to higher education. A-V Online should be considered a secondary source after first checking the AVLINE database. CD-ROM versions of the A-V Online database are distributed by SilverPlatter and Library Corporations.

Online Databases Including Audiovisuals

Three primary vendors provide access to databases that principally contain references to print information but also contain references to health sciences audiovisual materials: the National Library of Medicine (NLM), Bibliographic Retrieval Service (BRS), and DIALOG Information Services

(DIALOG). All of these services publish abbreviated instructions that give information about log-on and log-off procedures, system commands, and search features.

Three somewhat dated but still very useful publications describe how to limit searches to audiovisual materials. The first two are Van Camp's [2-3] search strategies for identifying audiovisual formats, which still apply to these same databases. The third, *Searching for Health Sciences Audiovisuals in Online Databases* [4], was designed for use in two half-day workshops. The first half of the textbook focuses on comprehensive searching techniques for AVLINE; the second half describes how to search the other health sciences databases containing audiovisual materials.

Online databases that contain reference to health science audiovisual materials include the following.

Agricola contains more than 1,000 audiovisual programs on nutrition education, diet therapy, and food technology and management.
Print Source: Catalog of the Food and Nutrition Information and Education Materials Center
Producer: Food and Nutrition Information and Education Materials Center, National Agricultural Library
Start Date and Update Frequency: 1973, monthly
Online Search Services: BRS: CAIN; DIALOG: File 10

Bioethicsline contains approximately 200 audiovisuals concerning the ethical aspect of health care and biomedical research.
Print Source: Bibliography of Bioethics
Producer: Center for Bioethics, Kennedy Institute of Ethics, Georgetown University
Start Date and Update Frequency: 1973, triannually
Online Search Service: MEDLARS

Combined Health Information Database (CHID) is a composite database of health information clearinghouses and databases produced by agencies within the U.S. Public Health Service and the Veterans Administration.
Print Source: Current Awareness in Health Education
Producer: Combined Health Information Database
Online Search Service: BRS: CHID

Child Abuse and Neglect contains more than 300 audiovisuals on the identification, prevention, treatment, and legal aspects of child abuse and neglect.
Print Source: Child Abuse and Neglect Audiovisual Materials

Producer: National Center on Child Abuse and Neglect
Start Date and Update Frequency: 1965, annually
Online Search Service: DIALOG: File 64

Computerized Aids Information Network (CAIN) contains audiovisuals on AIDS.
Producer: Los Angeles Gay and Lesbian Community Services Center
Online Search Service: General Videodex Corporation/DELPHI

Drug Info contains more than 200 films on educational, sociological, and psychological aspects of drug or alcohol use and abuse.
Producer: Drug Information Services, College of Pharmacy, University of Minnesota
Start Date and Update Frequency: 1968, infrequently
Online Search Service: BRS: DRUG

ERIC (Educational Resources Information Center) contains audiovisuals in all areas of education.
Print Sources: Resources in Education; Current Index to Journals in Education
Producer: ERIC Processing and Reference Facility
Start Date and Update Frequency: 1966, monthly
Online Search Services: BRS: ERIC; DIALOG: File 1

Exceptional Child Education Resources (ECER) contains audiovisuals on education of handicapped or gifted children and youth.
Print Source: Exceptional Child Education Abstracts
Producer: The Council for Exceptional Children
Start Date and Update Frequency: Audiovisuals added to file in 1977; monthly
Online Search Services: BRS: ECER; DIALOG: File 54

Family Resources Database (NCFR) contains more than 3,000 audiovisuals on all aspects of family relationships and services to families.
Producer: National Council on Family Relations
Start Date and Update Frequency: 1970, monthly
Online Search Services: BRS: NCFR; DIALOG: File 291; Executive Telecom System

Mental Health Abstracts contains more than 4,000 audiovisuals on mental health, mental illness, psychopharmacology, and personality.
Print Source: Selected Mental Health Audiovisuals
Producer: National Clearinghouse for Mental Health Information

Start Date and Update Frequency: 1969, monthly
Online Search Service: BRS: NCMH

OCLC (Online Computer Library Center) contains more than 23 million print and nonprint bibliographic records created by the cooperative efforts of libraries nationwide. Second to AVLINE, OCLC is the most comprehensive online reference tool available for audiovisual materials. More than 150 major health sciences libraries use the system to catalog their audiovisual and microcomputer collections. Recently the National Library of Medicine loaded the AVLINE tapes into the OCLC database, thereby enhancing the value of the database to libraries using OCLC to support health sciences audiovisual collection development, reference, and interlibrary loan services.

Several features make OCLC a major source for identifying bibliographic information on audiovisual and microcomputer software. A qualifier or media designator can be attached to a search for a known item or for a subject, thereby limiting the search to a media format. To limit the records retrieved to audiovisual materials, a search can be qualified with the value "med" which includes films, filmstrips, slides, videorecordings, and pictures. Sound recordings are limited by "rec" and computer files and software by "mrf."

Through OCLC's PRISM system, audiovisual and microcomputer titles in the OCLC database can be searched by title and subject or keywords. PRISM is a valuable system for cataloging materials, verifying bibliographic information, and identifying a loan source for known items.

For librarians who infrequently search OCLC, First Search may be the most efficient way to access the OCLC database. First Search is a menu-driven, user-friendly system that structures title and subject searches. Its ability to limit searches by format type and date make it relatively easy to identify current audiovisual and microcomputer materials.

Enhanced subject access to the OCLC database is available through OCLC's EPIC Service. Sophisticated search capabilities such as Boolean logic, keyword, and phrase searching make access to OCLC via EPIC the system of choice for a subject approach.

Rehabdata, or **NARIC,** contains approximately 200 audiovisuals on rehabilitation of the physically or mentally disabled. Subject areas include disability groups, such as the blind, deaf, developmentally disabled, spinal cord injured, and emotionally disturbed.

Producer: National Rehabilitation Information Center
Start Date and Update Frequency: 1965, monthly
Online Search Service: BRS: NRIC

Sport & Recreation contains about 400 audiovisuals on sports medicine, physical education, and recreation.
Print Source: Sport Bibliography
Producer: Sport Information Resources Center
Start Date and Update Frequency: 1975, quarterly
Online Search Service: SDC

Audiovisual Sourcebooks, Catalogs, and Guides

11.3 *National Library of Medicine Audiovisuals Catalog.* Bethesda, MD, National Library of Medicine, 1977- . 3 quarterly publications, annual cumulation.

11.4 *Guide to Locating Patient Education Audiovisual Materials.* McLean, VA, Health Sciences Communications Association, 1989.

11.5 *Patient Education Sourcebook Volume II.* McLean, VA, Health Sciences Communications Association, 1990.

11.6 *Educational Film & Video Locator.* 4th ed. New York, R. R. Bowker, 1990.

11.7 *The Video Source Book.* 13th ed. Detroit, MI, Gale, 1992.

National Library of Medicine Audiovisuals Catalog is a cumulation of citations to audiovisual materials and, since 1988, to microcomputer software cataloged by NLM. At present the catalog consists of three quarterly issues and the annual cumulation which is issued in lieu of a fourth quarterly. Audiovisual and microcomputer software cataloged for this publication is listed by MeSH descriptors and name or title. In addition, there is a comprehensive procurement source section providing the name, address, and telephone number of the media producers or distributors listed in the index. Changes to producer name, address, or telephone number are made in NLM's procurement record in the online Name Authority File (NAF) of the AVLINE database, making it an excellent source for current producer and distributor information.

A most useful feature of this catalog is the audiovisual serials index which appears as an appendix in each issue. This section is particularly useful because most libraries do not analyze audiovisual serials or provide full bibliographic cataloging in their in-house online catalogs to the individual titles of audiocassette, slidecassette, and videocassette serials. More than fifty audiovisual serials are indexed in this section, including the major serial collections such as Audio Digest, Network for Continuing Medical Education (NCME), and Johns Hopkins Medical Grand Rounds. New formats containing continuing medical education, such as video journals, are indexed in this section. From 1977 through 1983, the Audiovisual Serials Index was published as the *Index to Audiovisual Serials in the Health Sciences* by the Medical Library Association in cooperation with the National Library of Medicine.

Guide to Locating Patient Education Audiovisual Materials, compiled by the National Library of Medicine, provides comprehensive descriptions of various current sources and formats of information related to patient and consumer health information. In response to the growing need to identify instructional materials for health professionals providing patient education and for consumers concerned with preventive health care, NLM developed this guide to assist librarians, health professionals, and educators. The volume is organized into the following sections based on the format of the reference tool or the distribution source: books and journal articles; periodicals; directories and guides; databases; catalogs of loanable collections; commercial producers and distributors; and foundations, institutes, and other nonprofit organizations. Of particular importance is the chapter on online catalogs of patient education audiovisuals and patient education online source directories that include audiovisual materials. Most of these online sources have been discussed in the previous section.

Patient Education Sourcebook Volume II is a mediagraphic identification tool for patient education audiovisual programs. Most listings are videocassettes, 16mm films, slides, audiocassettes, videodiscs, or combinations of these formats. The majority of listings have been produced between 1985, the publication date of the first edition, and 1990. Volume I is no longer in print and has been updated by Volume II. More than 2,300 titles are described in the *Sourcebook,* which provides the production date and an abbreviation code for the producer. Descriptions of the programs are very brief. New to this edition is a foreign-language index. Although the majority of listings are for the English language, fourteen other languages are represented. Another new feature is the awards field, which indicates codes for major awards that programs have received.

The *Educational Film & Video Locator* has established itself as an indispensable reference tool for identifying audiovisual materials available for rent. As a listing of video and film titles held by the forty-six members of the Consortium of College and University Media Centers, the reference book is a unique compilation of their individual video and film collections. The fourth edition contains approximately 51,900 videos and films which were viewed and selected by library staffs in response to the requests of faculty supporting the curriculum. The records in this union list contain the abbreviation of the media centers that own the title. To facilitate the search process, five sections are provided: major subject groupings; subject headings and cross-index to subject; subject, title, and audience-level index; alphabetical list of film descriptions; and series listing. For programs that are not needed in permanent collections, cannot be borrowed on interlibrary loan, or are no longer available, this directory serves as a valuable source for identifying audiovisuals available for rent.

The Video Source Book is an important general audiovisual reference tool because of its extensive coverage. The 1992 two-volume edition and its supplement serve as a guide to approximately 126,000 programs currently available on video from more than 1,500 sources. Of the 450 subject headings used to classify videos, a significant number are related to health sciences disciplines. Although many entertainment titles are included in this volume, a significant number of training videos geared to patient and consumer health education are indexed. The program distributors section lists important information about the distributors described in the directory. Intended audience levels and a rating scale for most programs provide evaluative information. Descriptions of the programs are very brief, therefore once a title is identified, the librarian may need to consult producer or distributor catalogs and brochures for a full description.

Audiovisual Producers and Distributors

Locating the names and addresses of current producers and distributors of health sciences audiovisual materials cannot easily be done in one source. Collectively, the best sources would be the producer indexes of all the print catalogs and online databases described in this chapter. New and out-of-business companies can be easily identified by checking the producer and distributor indexes of the newly received editions of major audiovisual, microcomputer, and multimedia reference books against an in-house database of producer addresses. All of the reference tools described in this chapter, with the exception of the source described below, list the individual titles of programs as well as the names of the producers and distributors. If looking for producers' names and addresses only, along with information about audiovisual products and services, then the following directory will be helpful.

11.8 *AV Market Place 1993*. New Providence, NJ, R. R. Bowker, 1969- . Annual.

AV Market Place 1993 is a comprehensive directory of audio and video products, manufacturers, services, and suppliers in the United States and Canada. The 21st edition lists more than 1,300 products or services and 6,800 companies that supply them. The products, services and company index is organized by seven major categories: audio, audiovisual, computer systems, film, video, programming, and miscellaneous. This tool primarily describes categories of audiovisual services and products rather than audiovisual programs. Several of the additional sections of the directory contain valuable information unique to this source. For example, the "Reference Books" section contains an extensive list of major audiovisual reference materials that deal with such topics as audiovisual production techniques, multimedia education, audiovisual hardware, and software reviews. The "Associations" section identifies the major audiovisual trade associations, as well as selected media-related organizations and educational and library groups with an audiovisual interest.

Audiovisual Reviews

Published reviews of educational software are especially useful when they are written by an expert in the subject area covered by the audiovisual. By indicating the material's appropriateness for a specific use or audience level, a well-written media review can save time and money. Ratings or quotations from subject experts are helpful in determining the relative quality, the accuracy of the content, and currency of the program. Photocopies of reviews are also useful in promoting the use of learning resources materials in exhibits and in soliciting feedback from faculty on the suitability of the program to support the curriculum. Evaluative comments about the quality of the instructional design, content scope, presentation method, and production style are extremely valuable to the selection and collection development process.

Reviews published in health sciences journals are the most current and extensive source of evaluative information. Identifying the journals that publish reviews on audiovisual, microcomputer, and multimedia materials is a difficult task, because of the number of new and ceased journal titles and columns and the irregular frequency with which these reviews are published. A number of journal publications review audiovisual, microcomputer, and multimedia materials (Figure 11-2). This select list was compiled by first combining the journal sources noted in the 1988 edition of *Health Media Review Index* and HeSCA's 1989 *Guide to Locating Patient Education Audiovisual Materials*. Journal titles that had irregular and infrequent reviews columns were excluded from the list. Several new journal titles that review microcomputer and multimedia titles were then added.

11.9 *Media Profiles: The Health Science Edition*. West Park, NY, Olympic Media Information. Vol. 10- , 1984- . Quarterly, loose-leaf. Continues: *Hospital/Health Care Training Media Profiles*. Vols. 1-9, 1974-1983.

11.10 *Health Media Review Index 1984-86*. Metuchen, NJ, Scarecrow Press, 1988.

Media Profiles: The Health Science Edition continues to be one of the most informative review sources for health sciences audiovisuals. Reviews are

Figure 11-2. Journals Providing Reviews of Audiovisual, Microcomputer, and Multimedia Materials

AAOHN Journal
American Journal of Nursing
Anaesthesia
Annals of Emergency Medicine
AORN Journal
Birth: Issues in Perinatal Care and Education
Booklist
Choice
Circulation
Computer Applications in the Biosciences
Computer Methods and Programs in Biomedicine
Computers & Biomedical Research
Computers in Biology and Medicine
Computers in Healthcare
Computers in Nursing
Contemporary Drug Problems
Contemporary Psychology
Death Studies
Dental Assistant
Diabetes Care
Exceptional Children
Family Process
Feedback (HeSCA)
Geriatric Nursing
Gerontologist
Health Aims
Health Promotion
Heart and Lung: The Journal of Critical Care
Hospital and Community Psychiatry
Hospital Topics
Journal of AV Media in Medicine
Journal of Biocommunication
Journal of Clinical Child Psychology
Journal of Drug Issues
Journal of Gerontological Nursing
Journal of Nursing Staff Development
Journal of Nutrition Education
Journal of Rehabilitation
Journal of the American Dental Association
MD Computing
Media and Methods
Nursing Management
Nursing Outlook
Occupational Health and Safety
Physician and Sportsmedicine
Postgraduate Medicine
Public Health Reports
Respiratory Care
Software in Healthcare

written by health professionals and include separate sections for the content description, synopsis, and evaluation. Generally the reviews are fairly extensive, ranging from two to five columns of narrative comment. The evaluation section for each review is distinct from the content description and synopsis and includes a recommendation on the use of the materials and, when appropriate, any negative statements about the value of the program. Title and subject indexes using MeSH descriptors accompany each issue. A cumulative index exists for the first nine complete volumes, from 1974 to 1983, and for the next seven, volumes 10-17, 1984-1990. Content descriptions and synopses are usually more extensive than the actual program evaluations. Each issue now reviews approximately thirty titles, representing a small fraction of those produced.

Health Media Review Index is a guide to reviews and descriptions of commercially available audiovisual and microcomputer software for the medical, mental health, allied health, human resources, and related counseling professions. Reviews and program descriptions are collected and abstracted from reviews published in more than 130 health-related journals and audiovisual review sources. This edition includes abstracts of reviews and descriptions of more than 3,000 programs. The goal of *Health Media Review Index* was to complement other reference tools and not to duplicate existing sources. With this in mind, the guide did not include three major sources of audiovisual reviews and descriptions: AVLINE, *NLM Audiovisuals Catalog*, and Microcomputer Index and International Software Database. Of particular importance to this reference tool is the annotated list of health sciences journals whose reviews of audiovisual and microcomputer software were included in this guide. Librarians that want to keep abreast of current software reviews could regularly route these journals to the department responsible for audiovisual and microcomputer collection development. The source of each abstracted review is referenced in the title record, which enables the user to consult the original abstract for greater detail.

Media Festivals

Media festivals can be a prime source for identifying quality award-winning audiovisuals. Lists of the entries and winners are usually available from the media festival sponsor, and many are published in the association's newsletter. In 1988, McCalpin [5] identified more than forty organizations sponsoring health sciences nonprint media festivals or competitions. Section eight, entitled "Awards," lists organizations sponsoring health sciences media festivals or competitions in which recognition is given for entries in health categories. The media festivals are listed alphabetically, followed by a description of the purpose of the festival, the formats accepted and the scope of the contest, and the names of the awards.

In most cases, the titles of the winners of the festivals are noted and referenced to the full description of the program in the main section of the book. Media festival catalogs make excellent reference and collection development tools.

> 11.11 *HeSCA Media Festivals & Learning Resource Center Catalog.* McLean, VA, Health Sciences Communications Association, 1965- . Annual.
> 11.12 *Biennial John Muir Medical Center Film Festival: Catalog of Entries.* Walnut Creek, CA, John Muir Medical Center, 1976- . Biennial.

The HeSCA Media Festivals are one of the most significant international forums for recognizing and identifying current health sciences media. Now in its 17th year, the Festivals draw more than 300 entries annually. HeSCA Media Festivals offer five competitive festivals each year: film, interactive materials, print, still media, and video. Descriptions of all the materials submitted to the HeSCA Media Festivals, plus those that were accepted for the HeSCA Learning Resource Center, comprise the annual catalog. It is an excellent source for identifying audiovisual, microcomputer, and multimedia programs that were produced, released, or copyrighted the year preceding the festival.

The John Muir Medical Film Festival is an internationally recognized audiovisual media competition serving the needs of media producers, health professionals, educators, and consumers. Established in 1976 and held biennially since, the most recent catalog describes more than 600 entries on health and medical subjects from the United States and fifteen other countries. Audiovisual formats accepted for 1990 included film, 1/2-inch VHS videocassettes, and interactive videodiscs. Judges from the fields of media production, health care, and education selected 35 first-place winners, 45 second-place winners, and 155 finalists. The *Catalog of Entries* serves as an excellent reference tool because of the useful title, subject, and award winner indexes. More than 350 current names and addresses of producers and distributors are listed in the distribution companies index. The names of more than fifty other media festivals are also listed in the catalog. If a program has won other media festival awards, the abbreviations of those awards are also noted in the main record of the catalog. As a collection development tool, the catalog is very useful because it is first organized by thirty-five subject categories, which are then divided into two major sections: consumer entries and professional entries.

MICROCOMPUTER SOFTWARE AND COURSEWARE SOURCES

Print Catalogs, Directories, Indexes, and Guides

11.13 1993 *Healthcare CAI Directory.* Alexandria, VA, Stewart Publishing, 1986- . Annual.

11.14 *Software for Health Sciences Education: A Reference Catalog.* 4th ed. Ann Arbor, MI, University of Michigan Medical Center, 1993.

11.15 *Directory of Educational Software for Nursing.* 4th ed. New York, National League for Nursing, 1992. Biennial.

11.16 *Academic Courseware Exchange.* Santa Barbara, CA, Intellimation, 1990- . Semiannual.

11.17 *MD Computing.* New York, Springer-Verlag, 1983- . Bimonthly.

11.18 *Tools for Learning Courseware Catalog.* Milford, CT, IBM Academic Information Systems, 1990-91. Biennial.

11.19 *The Software Encyclopedia 1993: A Guide for Personal, Professional, and Business Users.* 8th ed. New Providence, NJ, R. R. Bowker, 1985- . Annual.

The *Healthcare CAI Directory* is one of the most comprehensive sources of microcomputer software programs available in the fields of medicine, dentistry, allied health, and veterinary medicine. Published annually, this directory is part of the interactive healthcare directory series that includes the publication year as part of the title. More than 460 current titles were described in this edition. Each entry includes the name and address of the producer, the subject of the program, audience level, a brief description or abstract of the program, the computer platform, and price. The producer/distributor index is a useful source for the current names, addresses, and phone numbers of health sciences CAI producers and serves as an excellent source for requesting catalogs and detailed brochures. Although the subject index is not detailed and contains only five broad subject groupings, it is useful in sorting out the dentistry, quiz/test banks, and programs eligible for CME credit. One of the directory's limitations is that it does not indicate the year in which programs were produced.

Software for Health Sciences Education now describes more than 500 computer programs for medical education. This new edition is one of the single most valuable reference tools because of its extensive coverage, interactive format, and comprehensive indexing. One of its unique features is that it is also distributed in an electronic format that can be loaded and searched on a Macintosh computer. Plans to make it available in a DOS format are underway. This capability enables specialized lists to be generated on demand, tailored to users' needs. Information on new programs was sought from health sciences professionals, educators, learning resource specialists, practicing physicians and nurses, and software producers. It is a particularly useful guide because each record includes a descriptive abstract along with hardware requirements, costs, and bibliographic data. All programs are cross-referenced by software type, subject area, target audience, vendor address, computer system, and educational credit. Subject access is a strong feature of this catalog because nearly 100 medical subject headings are used as indexing terms to describe the software. It is specific enough to research the availability of educational software within specific disciplines of medicine and the health sciences.

The *Directory of Educational Software for Nursing* provides extensive content descriptions and critical reviews for nearly 300 educational software programs for nursing. Program listings range from anatomy and physiology to nursing practice skills, patient care simulations, geriatrics, medical-surgical, maternity, pediatrics, and critical care. In addition, CAI tutorials for nursing research and administration are identified. New to this edition are reviews of more than forty interactive videodisc programs and indicators of decision-making levels for simulations. As a selection tool and faculty guide to selecting quality courseware, this resource is invaluable because the titles are evaluated by health professionals. Several accompanying narrative sections provide useful information about evaluating CAI and interactive videodisc programs and on rating decision-making levels.

The *Academic Courseware Exchange*, formerly published by Kinko's Service Corporation, is an excellent source for Macintosh educational software. Published twice annually, the catalog keeps abreast of current Macintosh courseware geared to higher education. More than 70% of the titles formerly distributed by Kinko's were incorporated in the new edition. Intellimation now distributes more than 200 unique courseware programs, including a few CD-ROM and IVD titles. To conform to the academic computing environment, most of the programs can run on a network and offer site license agreements. Subject areas of particular importance to the health sciences are anatomy, physiology, clinical chemistry, microbiology, nutrition, hematology, immunology, and statistics.

MD Computing is the official journal of the American Medical Informatics Association. It serves as a current and comprehensive source for detailed information on more than 1,200 microcomputer software and hardware products within the medical field, including nursing and dental informatics. Annually, the November/December issue is devoted to a medical hardware and software buyers' guide, and the July/August issue publishes the annual directory of medical hardware and software companies. The buyers' guide is first organized by subject categories ranging from AIDS to word processing, where medical subject headings are interspersed with hardware terms. Company names and addresses and the products they distribute are then described within each subject category. Two accompanying indexes facilitate the use of the buyers' guide: one lists the subject categories and one lists the companies and the products they have included. This guide is especially useful in identifying producers and distributors by a medical subject approach. Broad subject categories such as graduate medical education, nursing education, and gynecology, as well as specific subject access such as diabetes mellitus, smoking, and hypothermia make it easy to identify materials by subject. Various kinds of software applications—ranging from computer assisted instruction to information management tools, library systems, and office management packages—are described in this guide. Specific titles of software packages are referenced and annotated.

Tools for Learning Courseware Catalog was compiled by IBM Academic Information Systems to bring together instructional software for higher education that run on IBM systems. The purpose of the catalog is to help promote software available to faculty. Organized according to academic disciplines for easy reference, this edition describes more than 450 individual offerings. Entries for each title include a brief abstract based on information provided by the author or publisher, as well as pertinent technical data and ordering and price information. Subject areas that are of particular interest to the health sciences include computer science, biology, environmental science, dentistry, medicine, nursing, nutrition, pharmacology, and physiology. Interspersed throughout the catalog are a few interactive videodisc programs. Many of the programs are distributed by Wisc-Ware, Academic Computing Center, University of Wisconsin.

The Software Encyclopedia was developed to provide detailed information on microcomputer software for personal, professional, and business use. Software that could support an informatics curriculum or information management program are described within this catalog. Business applications such as databases that manage patient records, medical dictionaries that can run in conjunction with word processors, treatment and diagnosis expert systems, and medical clip art are included for each major computer type.

The eighth edition contains entries for more than 16,000 microcomputer software packages from more than 4,000 publishers. Software products are arranged first by system compatibility, then by specific application. Subject areas of particular interest to the health sciences and libraries under the broad subject heading of medicine include accounting, anesthesiology, chiropractic, database management, dental, dental office management, dictionaries, education, fitness, graphics, hospital management, nursing home management, ophthalmology, orthodontics, pathology, pediatrics, pharmacy, psychiatry, and radiology.

Computer applications that would be useful in managing library records or systems such as media booking and scheduling programs, integrated library systems, LAN and hard disk management software, and telecommunications packages are interspersed throughout the catalog. Updated annually, this tool is a valuable resource for microcomputer lab managers, information technology staff, and faculty supporting computer applications in medicine and health.

Online Databases for Microcomputer Software

Online sources of information about microcomputer hardware and software would be the reference tool of choice because of currency and enhanced searching capabilities. At the present time, only one online database provides access to bibliographic descriptions of health sciences education software exclusively. The Health Sciences Libraries Consortium, Computer Based Learning (HSLC CBL) database is becoming the most comprehensive source for medical education courseware information. It is accessible via the Internet at no charge and invites libraries and the health sciences community to contribute software records on a daily basis. Three other valuable sources differ in scope. *Microcomputer Index* describes references to the journal literature about microcomputers and educational technology. Microcomputer Software Guide describes software programs in all subject areas. SOFT describes information about microcomputer products and services. Although the latter three resources are very useful for information about the broad fields of computer science and information technology, other online sources that cover print and audiovisual materials, mentioned earlier in this chapter, may be more resourceful and economical when conducting a subject search on medical and health sciences topics. The HSLC CBL database, OCLC, and AVLINE are the recommended systems to search first before querying the more expensive BRS and DIALOG databases.

11.20 *Health Sciences Libraries Consortium, Computer Based Learning.* Philadelphia, PA, Health Sciences Libraries Consortium, 1987- . Daily.

11.21 *Microcomputer Index.* Medford, NJ, Learned Information, 1981- . Monthly.

11.22 *Microcomputer Software Guide.* New York, R. R. Bowker, 1988- . Monthly.

11.23 *SOFT.* Weston, CT, Online, 1988- . Monthly. Produces: *Online Microcomputer Software Guide and Directory.*

Health Sciences Libraries Consortium, Computer Based Learning database originally included about seventy descriptions of health sciences computer programs that were developed with grant funds. The database, begun in 1987, contains listings of IBM-compatible and Macintosh programs used in health sciences education. The project was endorsed and funded by the Education Working Group of the American Medical Informatics Association (AMIA). Records have also been contributed by the University of Michigan's 1993 edition of *Software for Health Sciences Education*. Of particular value to users searching the database is the user-friendly interface and the ability to use Boolean logic. NISO standards of searching were incorporated. Instructions for searching the database are provided online. The database is currently searchable through HSLC HealthNET, the consortium's online system used by more than 250 medical schools, hospitals, and libraries in Pennsylvania, Delaware, New Jersey, and New York. Through AMIA grant funds, the HSLC has made this database accessible to all via the Internet's Telnet protocol. The HSLC CBL database can be accessed by telnetting to [hslc.org]. When the system asks for a USERNAME prompt, type [CBL].

Microcomputer Index, a database distributed by DIALOG as file 233, contains abstracts and citations to literature on the use of microcomputers in business, education, and the home. The publications covered index articles of many types, including software and hardware reviews, product announcements, buyer and vendor guides, company news items, and book reviews. Software review coverage was expanded to include library, chemistry, engineering, and medical applications. The database indexes more than eighty English-language journals and corresponds to the print publication *Microcomputer Index*.

Microcomputer Software Guide, a database distributed by DIALOG as file 278, contains information on microcomputer software programs available or produced in the United States. The database is used to produce the Bowker publication *Software Encyclopedia*. Source data are derived from information received directly from more than 4,000 software publishers as well as industry sources, such as press releases, periodicals, and books. More than 35,000 records comprise the database, where approximately 500 new records are added each month. Although this database is comprehensive for sources of business software, many of the producers of educational software, especially from academic institutions, do not participate in submitting bibliographic and purchasing information.

SOFT, a database distributed by BRS and DIALOG, contains current business and professional microcomputer software product descriptions plus related information on costs, applications, hardware requirements, documentation availability, operating environment specifications, and other software used with the package. Critical review information is included as well as a short abstract. The file is selective and lists the best and most significant software in business, finance, library and information science, life sciences, professional applications, science, and systems and utilities.

Educational Software Awards

Exemplary educational software can be identified by the winners of educational media festivals. One of the highest honors an author of instructional software can receive is the best software or distinguished software designation in the annual EDUCOM/NCRIPTAL Higher Education Software Awards Competition. EDUCOM is a nonprofit consortium of nearly 600 colleges and universities concerned with computing and related technology in education. NCRIPTAL, the National Center for Research to Improve Postsecondary Teaching and Learning, is funded jointly by the University of Michigan and the U.S. Department of Education. Winners of EDUCOM's Software and Curriculum Innovation Awards are published annually in EDUCOM's *Educational Use of Information Technology (EUIT)* newsletter, accessible through Internet at the following address: EUITNews@EDUCOM.BICNIC.EDU. IBM Academic Information Systems published a special edition to the *Tools for Learning Courseware Catalog* (*see* 11.18) describing all the software that runs on IBM systems honored in the competition. Another good source for award winning health sciences educational software is the HeSCA Media Festivals. HeSCA's Interactive Media Festival evaluates CAI and interactive videodisc programs geared to higher education curriculum and continuing medical education.

MULTIMEDIA REFERENCE SOURCES

A multimedia workstation is one that provides substantially more sensory content in the human interface than a traditional computer workstation. This increased sensory content includes the use of still image, motion video, color, increased resolution, and audio [6]. Interactive videodisc materials are considered to be a multimedia format because they integrate various formats of text, video, and audio information, and they require specialized hardware and additional peripherals to operate. Ullmer [7] defines the key instrumental ingredients of interactive technology to be microcomputers, optical disc systems, input and display devices, and software programs for authoring and delivering instructional programs. The key conceptual ingredients that underlie instructional program development are the consolidation of information resources on disc media, multimedia presentation, the individualization of instructional delivery, and most importantly, interactivity and adaptivity in lesson design.

Multimedia titles are also being delivered by way of CD-ROM formats, with only about four dozen titles available as of early 1992 [8]. By far, reference and educational multimedia programs are the most common. Illustrations in the new multimedia program Animated Dissection of Anatomy for Medicine (ADAM) are stored in a CD-ROM format. Several medical clip art packages are also being distributed in a CD-ROM format because of the random access and rapid retrieval features of CD-ROM technology.

Multimedia Catalogs, Directories, and Guides

11.24 *1993 Healthcare Videodisc Directory.* Alexandria, VA, Stewart Publishing, 1986- . Annual.

11.25 *1993 Healthcare CD-ROM Directory.* Alexandria, VA, Stewart Publishing, 1990- . Annual.

11.26 *Multimedia Applications for Health Sciences Curricula.* Milford, CT, IBM Academic Information Systems, 1991.

11.27 *Videodiscs at the National Library of Medicine.* Bethesda, MD, National Library of Medicine, 1992.

11.28 *Proceedings of the Symposium on Computer Applications in Medical Care.* New York, American Medical Informatics Association; Mc-Graw-Hill, 1976- . Annual.

11.29 *Videodisc Compendium for Education and Training.* St. Paul, MN, Emerging Technology Consultants, 1988- .

The *1993 Healthcare Videodisc Directory* has been published annually for over five years and continues to be one of the single most valuable sources for identifying health sciences interactive videodisc materials. The title of the catalog changes annually when the new publication year is inserted as the first word in the title. More than 475 unique titles are described in the catalog, 141 of them new, and approximately 90% are available for purchase. Those titles not available for distribution, primarily from academic settings, are included to allow readers to network with other educators who are involved in the development of videodisc programs in their areas of interest. In an effort to overcome the hardware barrier, many programs now are being offered for multiple configurations. The most common configuration is InfoWindow-compatible, with more than 30% of the programs available. Seventeen percent of the titles are available for the two-screen Macintosh platform. Representing a new trend in educational technology, nearly sixty titles take advantage of the relatively new laser barcode system. The preface contains a brief but informative definition of the seven interactive hardware configurations.

1993 Healthcare CD-ROM Directory is just one of a three-book set of interactive healthcare directories published by Stewart Publishing that have become a primary source for locating interactive videodisc, CAI, and

CD-ROM materials in the health sciences. Although the vast majority of titles in the *CD-ROM Directory* contains citations to medical literature and databases, there also are more than a dozen educational programs included. As the evolution of storing graphic images moves from analog to digital, more educational software programs will be produced in this format. The subject areas that have utilized this technology to great advantage so far are anatomy and physiology because of the large number of still frame images and the capability of incorporating sound. The program descriptions are fairly detailed and hardware requirements and purchasing information are complete. The introductory chapter on compact disc technology is very helpful in clarifying the differences between the seven CD-ROM formats and platforms.

Multimedia Applications for Health Sciences Curricula is a thirty-one page catalog that describes IBM multimedia programs that were developed by the Health Care Interactive Videodisc Consortium. To identify programs geared to either the basic sciences or clinical sciences, the catalog utilizes a Knowledge Base Matrix as a guide for curriculum developers seeking to apply multimedia applications to enhance basic course offerings at health sciences institutions. Each program is indicated by its use—instruction, research, or clinical—as well as its suitability for curricula in schools of medicine, nursing, or allied health. The contact directory identifies where these applications solutions can be acquired.

Videodiscs at the National Library of Medicine describes 104 health sciences videodisc programs that either appear in the AVLINE database or are available for demonstration in The Learning Center (TLC) of the Educational Technology Branch of NLM. System requirements, credits, and abstracts are provided for each program. For libraries with various interactive videodisc systems and levels of videodisc equipment, the indexes are very useful in identifying level I, II, and III videodisc programs. Videodiscs available for Macintosh systems and videodisc programs accessible by barcode reader are described in separate indexes. Updated lists of NLM's videodisc holdings can be created by searching the subheading "videodiscs (SH)" on AVLINE.

The *Proceedings of the Symposium on Computer Applications in Medical Care (SCAMC)* is an excellent source for identifying newly produced multimedia and courseware materials within the medical specialties. SCAMC is a conference sponsored by the American Medical Informatics Association and its published proceedings can serve as a selection tool. Two- to four-page articles describe how clinical simulations, multimedia programs, and clinical applications were developed and implemented in an academic or hospital setting. This publication may be one of the few sources that can identify software under development that may never reach the commercial sector.

Videodisc Compendium for Education and Training describes more than 2,200 titles from more than 240 producers of laserdiscs, CDs, and multimedia software on a broad range of topics, including health care. The broad subject area of health is further subdivided by care, children at risk, medical, and safety. The catalog is produced in a journal-like format. Descriptions of the software are brief but informative. Useful acquisitions information, such as the producer's phone number, is noted within the record. Names and addresses of organizations that serve the laserdisc industry and publications that dedicate a portion of their publication to laserdisc technology are listed.

Conferencing Networks

11.30 *E.T. Net (Educational Technology Network).* Bethesda, MD, National Library of Medicine, 1991- .

E.T. Net is an online computer conference network that electronically links developers and users of interactive technology in health sciences education [9]. Conceived to aid health sciences educators faced with a lack of available information on interactive courseware, it uses advanced computer conferencing software especially designed to facilitate online discussions. E.T. Net consists of subject matter message areas called "conferences." These conferences are asynchronous message areas, rather than live, online, real-time interactions. Current conferences are AVLINE, CAI, shareware, hardware, digital images, UMLS Users, NUCARE, and general. E.T. Net allows users and developers to share reviews on software, hardware, and videodiscs, as well as new applications of interactive hardware in health sciences education. Sponsored by the Educational Technology Branch of the Lister Hill National Center for Biomedical Communications, E.T. Net is open to professionals engaged in either the development or use of interactive technology in health professions education and nursing care research. It is available at no cost, twenty-four hours a day, seven days a week. The user may interact with E.T. Net through user-friendly menus. E.T. Net is accessed through the Internet or a local SprintNet number. For Canada, DATAPAC access is available. If these services are unavailable, contact the Learning Center for Interactive Technology at the Lister Hill National Center for Biomedical Communications at (301) 496-0508.

Hardware and Educational Technology Sources

11.31 *The Directory of Multimedia Equipment, Software and Services.* 2nd ed. Fairfax, VA, International Communications Industries Association, 1992- . Annual.

11.32 *The Directory of Video, Computer, and Audio-Visual Products.* 38th ed. Fairfax, VA, International Communications Industries Association, 1955- . Annual.

11.33 *Multimedia Computing in the Health Science Library.* Chapel Hill, NC, Health Sciences Consortium, 1992.

11.34 *Multimedia Product Guide from IBM.* Atlanta, GA, IBM Corporation, Multimedia Information Center, 1993.

11.35 *Multimedia: Getting Started.* Cupertino, CA, Apple Computer, 1991.

11.36 *Multimedia Source Guide: Supplement to T.H.E. Journal.* Tustin, CA, T.H.E. Journal, 1992-93.

The *Directory of Multimedia Equipment, Software and Services* is a new major 500-page publication covering the entire range of multimedia technology. Its primary focus is to describe multimedia hardware. Listings for equipment, software, and services in the directory are accepted from the manufacturer, producer, service provider, or from the sole distributor of such products and services. All of the products must be currently available on the market. Of particular value to those selecting hardware are the photographs of each product along with the technical description and retail price. Five major sections are included in the directory: consultants and services, production tools, hardware and peripherals, multimedia systems, and videodisc and CD-ROM titles. Several short articles published in the introduction provide a good overview of the following topics: selecting computer-video interfaces; CD-ROM; fiber and video; LCD technology; and multimedia authoring tools. Of particular value to those selecting software is the multimedia awards showcase, which lists the winners of seven major multimedia festivals. Coverage of multimedia titles is not very extensive, however, the photographs of the software package or sample screens from the program provide some unique information. The format of the directory is very similar to the familiar *Directory of Video, Computer and Audio-Visual Products* because it is also published by the International Communications Industries Association (ICIA).

The *Directory of Video, Computer, and Audio-Visual Products* is an annual publication compiled by the ICIA, the trade association of the communications technologies industry, formerly the National Audio-Visual Association. Product information is contributed by the manufacturers. The directory goes further than just providing product information on audiovisual, computer, and video hardware; it also includes manufacturers, producers, professionals, and dealers who help users find product information. Complete information for more than 2,000 equipment items, including specifications, photographs, and prices, is provided. Entries are classified by type of equipment and then arranged alphabetically by proprietary name. Other pertinent information includes model number; physical description; accessories; and notes indicating special features, available modifications, or ordering specifics. Although the directory claims to be a comprehensive source, not all models and manufacturers are included, because listings are submitted by the manufacturer rather than compiled by the publisher.

Multimedia Computing in the Health Science Library is a practical guide to creating an integrated computing environment to support the use of multimedia materials and information systems. The series of seven articles is a case study and cookbook for building and managing a computer lab in a health sciences environment following the Integrated Advanced Information Management System(IAIMS) model established by the National Library of Medicine.

Multimedia Product Guide is a booklet published by IBM describing its Ultimedia product lines and multimedia solutions available from IBM. Although it only references to IBM products, it is still very useful in making technical distinctions between various models of computers and monitors. In addition, it includes product information about authoring systems and tools, courseware and applications, multimedia complementary products, multimedia programs, multimedia classes, and Ultimedia apparel.

Multimedia: Getting Started is a glossy guide that provides an introduction to the technology that underlies integrating multimedia into teaching. The narrative includes a technical overview of multimedia technology written in a simplistic style. Graphic illustrations and photographs provide excellent visual explanations of technical concepts. Topics covered include multimedia technology, the basics of sound, digitized audio, CD audio, graphics for multimedia, graphics scanners, the basics of videodisc, color displays, digital videodisc, and developing multimedia.

Multimedia Source Guide: Supplement to T.H.E. Journal is a primer on what the various components to a multimedia hardware system are and how they are used. It is not a technical reference manual or an exhaustive compilation of products that could in some way be labeled multimedia. Rather the directory listings comprise those packages and hardware descriptions deemed best suited to educational needs and environments. It is divided into nine categories: whole development or delivery platforms; software and courseware; players; presentation devices; video/graphic input devices; add-in cards; output devices; mass storage devices; and multimedia publishers, distributors, and services.

REFERENCES

1.Hannigan G, Brown J. Managing public access microcomputers in health sciences libraries. Chicago: Medical Library Association, 1990.

2. Van Camp A. Health sciences audiovisuals in online databases. Database 1980 Sept;3:17-27.

3. Van Camp A. Health sciences audiovisuals in online databases. Part 2. Database 1982 Sept;5(3):23-39.

4. Foxman D, Jacobs A, Watson L, Van Camp A. Searching for health sciences audiovisuals in online databases. Baltimore, MD: Southeastern/Atlantic Regional Medical Library Services, 1984.

5. McCalpin D. Health media review index 1984-86. Metuchen, NJ: Scarecrow Press, 1988;627-55.

6. Champine G. MIT Project Athena: a model for distributed campus computing. Bedford, MA: Digital Press, 1991.

7. Ullmer E. Interactive technology. Bethesda, MD: National Library of Medicine, 1990. Lister Hill Monograph, 90-92.

8. Stewart S. Healthcare CD-ROM directory. Alexandria, VA: Stewart Publishing, 1992.

9. E.T. Net Fact Sheet. Bethesda, MD: Lister Hill National Center for Biomedical Communications, National Library of Medicine, 1992 Feb.

READINGS

Abbey L. Dental Informatics: integrating technology into the dental environment. New York: Springer-Verlag, 1991.

Ball MJ, Hannah KJ, Jelger UG, Peterson H, eds. Nursing informatics: where caring and technology meet. New York: Springer-Verlag, 1989.

Branyan-Broadbent B, Wood R, eds. Educational media and technology yearbook. Volume 18. Englewood, CO: Libraries Unlimited, Association for Educational Communications and Technology, 1992.

Chao J. Continuing medical education software: a comparative review. J Fam Pract 1992 May;34(5):598-604.

Kander M. Healthcare video directory: an educational resource for healthcare practitioners and administrators. Owings Mill, MD: National Health Pub., 1988.

Updegrove N. Adult/patient education materials. Beltsville, MD: U.S. Department of Agriculture. National Agricultural Library, 1990.

Weal E. Creating and managing an academic computer lab. Sunnyvale, CA: PUBLIX Information Products, for Apple Computer, 1991.

CHAPTER 12

Medical and Health Statistics

Frieda Weise and Judith Johnson

Health statistics encompass a highly interdisciplinary area of medical reference and represent challenges to the librarian that may be unique in the field. Rarely will such an array of reference tools and such an opportunity for frustration be found. Today's medical librarian can characterize the most obscure syndromes or provide toxicity data for a list of compounds that seems to grow exponentially, yet the same librarian may be forced into a posture of defeat when asked to produce a seemingly obvious statistic. There is no shortage of statistical reference material available. Difficulties in locating the needed data stem more from fragmented and uncoordinated data collection efforts, which result in little or no data for some topics and duplication for other topics [1]. Variations in coverage—geographical areas, time periods, methods of data collection and analysis, sample size, and definitions of categories—are common among data collection agencies. Nevertheless, library patrons expect consistent reporting and reliable comparisons.

A successful search is hampered still further by a lack of adequate subject access through indexes and the time lag in publication of data. While the statistics seeker requires specifics, subject access is limited due to the multiplicity of numbers that can appear in one table. Finally, most statistics are out of date long before they are published; for example, most 1980 census data were published after 1983.

All of the problems associated with the location of statistics would be inconsequential if health-related statistics and the demands placed upon them were not so important. Such statistics exist to provide planners, administrators, and researchers with a comprehensive picture of the nation's health. Statistics can be used to shed light on various aspects of the population, to understand how health services and health programs are being used, to evaluate the effectiveness of health care delivery, and to identify the country's health care needs.

Health statistics include a wide spectrum of information: vital statistics (birth, death, marriage, and divorce); morbidity and other measures of health status; health care facilities, manpower, and education; use of health care services; and health care costs and expenditures. For these statistics to be meaningful, however, they must also be linked to population and demographic data.

Among the important demographic characteristics are geographic distribution, age, sex, race, and marital status, and socioeconomic characteristics such as ethnicity, income, education, and employment. Population characteristics are often correlated with health statistics in the hope of discovering some cause and effect. For example, why is the incidence of a disease higher among one ethnic group than another? Why does the infant mortality rate differ between races and socioeconomic groups? The librarian's task, however, is usually to find the basic information in these questions—the incidence of the disease or the infant mortality rate—a formidable task in itself.

TERMINOLOGY

The terminology used in the area of health statistics is not as extensive as in many other disciplines in the health sciences. There is surprisingly little jargon that only an insider would be able to decipher. However, it is helpful to keep the definitions of some of the most frequently occurring terms in mind when trying to locate statistical information. The search strategy and outcome of the search for a statistic may depend on one's understanding of some very basic terms. The following definitions are based on those found in *Discursive Dictionary of Health Care* [2] and *Dictionary of Epidemiology,* first and second editions [3].

In reviewing the definitions it becomes apparent that *rate* is a very important term in health statistics. Rate appears in connection with terms such as natality, mortality, incidence, and prevalence. As noted in the definitions, rate expresses the number of events occurring during a specified period of time within a particular population. For example, it is meaningless to say there were thirty-three cases of measles in Chicago without knowing the time period during which they occurred and the population within which they occurred. A rate will express this concept. Stating that the incidence rate of measles in Chicago was 11 per 1,000 children aged 6 years and under during the 4-week period ending November 30, 1982, will give an indication of the real magnitude of the disease.

Table 12-1. Frequently Occurring Terms

Acute disease	A disease that is characterized by a single episode of fairly short duration from which the patient returns to his or her normal or previous state and level of activity. While acute diseases are frequently distinguished from chronic diseases, there is no standard definition or distinction. It is worth noting that an acute episode of a chronic disease (e.g., an episode of diabetic coma in a patient with diabetes) is often treated as an acute disease.
Biometry	The application of statistical methods to the study of numerical data based on biological observations and phenomena.
Chronic disease	A disease that has one or more of the following characteristics: is permanent; leaves residual disability; is caused by nonreversible pathological alteration; requires special training of the patient for rehabilitation; or may be expected to require a long period of supervision, observation, or care.
Cohort study	An inquiry in which a group is chosen for the presence of a specific characteristic at or during a specified time and followed over time for the appearance of particular related characteristics.
Communicable disease	An illness due to a specific infectious agent or its toxic products that arises through transmission of that agent or its products from an infected person, animal, or reservoir to a susceptible host. These diseases are also known as "infectious diseases."
Demography	The study of populations, especially with reference to size and density, fertility, growth, age distribution, migration, and vital statistics, and the interaction of all these with social and economic conditions.
Epidemic	The occurrence in a community or region of cases of an illness, specific health-related behavior, or other health-related events clearly in excess of normal expectancy. The term may also be used to describe outbreaks of disease in animal or plant population.
Epidemiology	The study of the distribution and determinants of

Table 12-1 (continued)

	health-related states or events in specified populations, and the application of this study to the control of health problems.
Ethnic group	A social group characterized by a distinctive social and cultural tradition that is maintained within the group from generation to generation, a common history and origin, and a sense of identification with the group. Members of the group have distinctive features in their way of life, shared experiences, and often a common genetic heritage.
Health facilities	Collectively, all buildings and facilities used in the provision of health services. Usually limited to facilities that are built for the purpose of providing health care, such as hospitals and nursing homes, and thus, not including office buildings for physicians' offices.
Health manpower	Collectively, all men and women working in the provision of health services whether as individual practitioners or employees of health institutions and programs, whether or not professionally trained, and whether or not subject to public regulation. Facilities and manpower are the principal health resources used in producing health services.
Health resources	Resources (human, monetary, or material) used in producing health care and services. They include money, health manpower, health facilities, equipment, and supplies.
Health status	Measures of the nature and extent of diseases, disability, discomfort, attitudes, and knowledge concerning health, and of the perceived need for health care. Health status measures identify groups in need of, or at risk of needing, services.
Incidence rate	A rate expressing the number of new events or new cases of a disease in a defined population at risk, within a specified period of time; it is a measure of the number of "attacks" of a disease or condition during a particular time. The term incidence is sometimes used to express "incidence rates."

Table 12-1 (continued)

Incubation period	The time interval between invasion by an infectious agent and appearance of the first sign or symptom of the disease in question.
Life table	A summarizing technique used to describe the pattern of mortality and survival in populations. The survival data are time specific and cumulative probabilities of survival of a group of individuals subject, throughout life, to the age-specific death rates in question.
Morbidity	Any departure, subjective or objective, from a state of physiological or psychological well-being. In this sense, sickness, illness, and morbid condition are similarly defined and synonymous. Morbidity is usually stated in terms of incidence rate and prevalence rate.
Mortality rate	An estimate of the proportion of a population that dies during a specified period. Also referred to as the death rate.
Natality rate	A rate expressing the number of live births in a given year.
Notifiable disease	A disease that, by statutory requirements, must be reported to the public health authority in the pertinent jurisdiction (federal, state, or local) when the diagnosis is made. A disease deemed of sufficient importance to the public health to require that its occurrence be reported to health authorities, such as a sexually transmitted disease. Notifiable diseases are generally communicable diseases.
Population	The number of inhabitants of a given country or area; but also, in sampling, the whole collection of units from which a sample may be drawn; not necessarily a population of persons; the units may be institutions, records, or events. The sample is intended to give results that are representative of the whole population.
Prevalence rate	The total number of all individuals who have an attribute or disease at a particular time (or during a particular period) divided by the population at risk of having the attribute or disease at this point in time or midway through the period.

Table 12-1 (continued)

Utilization rate	A rate measuring the use of a single service or type of service, e.g., hospital care, physician visits, prescription drugs. Use is expressed in rates per unit of population at risk for a given period, e.g., number of admissions to a hospital per 1,000 persons per year.
Vital statistics	Systematically tabulated information concerning births, marriages, divorces, separations, and deaths based on registrations of these vital events.

The general formula to express rates is

$$\frac{\text{Number of events (deaths, disease, etc.) in a specified period of time}}{\text{population at risk of experiencing the event}} \quad \text{X 1,000 or 100,000} = \text{incidence rate}$$

The multiplier of 1,000 or 100,000 is used to produce a rate that is a manageable whole number [4].

If, in the case of Chicago, 33 cases of measles are reported during November among a population of 3,000 children aged 6 years and under, the formula to arrive at the incidence rate of 11 per 1,000 children is

$$\frac{\text{33 (cases during November)}}{\text{3,000 (population at risk)}} \quad \text{X 1,000} = 11 \text{ (incidence rate)}$$

The librarian must also be aware of the implications of the terms *incidence* and *prevalence* as they relate to data collection of infectious and chronic diseases. Confusion regarding incidence rates and prevalence rates can lead to very frustrating experiences for the searcher, because rarely, if ever, are incidence statistics available for chronic diseases. The long-term nature of chronic disease makes it difficult to determine the exact onset of a disease such as alcoholism, which is the primary piece of information needed for incidence statistics. People with chronic diseases, in fact, may not contact their physicians until an acute complication of the disease manifests itself. Even prevalence statistics may be difficult to locate for chronic diseases, because these are not notifiable diseases. Only infectious diseases are reportable by law to the Centers for Disease Control; no one agency has continuing responsibility for collection of statistics on all diseases.

AGENCIES AND ORGANIZATIONS

If data collection is uncoordinated and no one agency is responsible for all kinds of health statistics, how does anyone find anything? An awareness of which agencies and organizations collect which health statistics and a familiarity with their publications can serve not only as an aid in finding an answer in a published source, but also as a means of obtaining information about what has been or will be published. A telephone call to the appropriate organization can save hours of frustration and searching for data that may not be available.

In any discussion of the production of health statistics, it is important to keep a few points in mind. First, the data collection system is decentralized—it reflects the organization of the health care system in the United States. There are many government agencies—federal, state, and local—involved, as well as private organizations.

Second, collecting health statistics is a relatively new activity in the United States. The U. S. Constitution provided for a decennial census (since 1790) to apportion congressional representation from each state, but the need for vital and other health statistics was not recognized at the time the nation was founded. Therefore, collecting this data did not develop as a national undertaking, but rather first as a local, then state, and eventually a national function. For example, it was not until 1933 that all forty-eight states and the District of Columbia participated in the national birth and death registration program, and it was not until 1925 that reports on notifiable diseases were received from all states [5]. To carry the point still further, it was not until 1956 that Congress enacted the legislation to establish the U.S. National Health Survey within the Public Health Service to produce statistics on disease, injury, impairment, disability, and related topics [6].

Third, data collection is very expensive. Although there may be a statistic for every topic, it may, in fact, not have been collected by any agency because there was no perceived program need. Utility of the end products of data collection is an important consideration when expenditures for gathering statistics are involved.

This brief discussion points out a few of the reasons why agencies or organizations collect health statistics in the way that they do. It would not be practical to describe here all the agencies and organizations involved in health statistics collection activities; consequently, the following discussion covers those most heavily involved. The publications of these agencies are generally primary sources; that is, the data were collected, analyzed, and published by the agency. Agency publications are also sometimes secondary sources and will generally note the original source of the data.

Government Agencies

The primary responsibility for the collection and dissemination of health statistics in the United States rests with various agencies in the Department of Health and Human Services. Organized in 1960, the National Center for Health Statistics (NCHS) is the principal agency which "collects, analyzes, and disseminates health statistics on vital events and health activities to reflect the people's health status, health needs, and health resources" [7]. This is done principally through a national vital registration system covering births, deaths, marriages, and divorces; by a series of continuing surveys of the ambulatory and institutionalized population; and by surveys of health facilities. The two major publications containing vital statistics are the *Monthly Vital Statistics Report* (see 12.11) and the annual *Vital Statistics of the United States* (see 12.10).

The *Vital and Health Statistics Series* (see 12.12) contains published results of such surveys as the National Health Interview Survey, the National Health Examination Survey, the Hospital Discharge Survey, and the National Ambulatory Medical Care Survey, among others. All of the surveys taken together constitute the National Health Survey.

Advance Data (see 12.13) is a continuing series of reports published as a means for early release of data from NCHS surveys and collection. More detailed versions of these surveys later appear in one of the *Vital and Health Statistics Series*.

The Centers for Disease Control (CDC) protect "the public health of the Nation by providing leadership and direction in the prevention and control of diseases and other preventable conditions and responding to public health emergencies" [8], including, for example, childhood lead-based paint poisoning, urban rat control, and vector-borne disease. As the incidence of many known communicable diseases has declined, CDC's programs have been expanded to include noncommunicable diseases. Data on notifiable diseases are collected and published weekly in the *MMWR: Morbidity and Mortality Weekly Report* (see 12.14). The CDC also publishes considerable statistical material in its *Surveillance Summaries* (see 12.16), now published quarterly as part of the *MMWR*. Included in the surveillance program are such topics as abortion, congenital malformations, and diabetes.

In addition to its statistical activities, CDC carries out regulatory activities, such as monitoring laboratory standards, evaluating occupational health hazards, and preventing imported diseases. These statements are presented in its *Recommendations and Reports* (*see* 12.17), published irregularly as part of the *MMWR*.

As the agency responsible for the federal government's two major health care financing programs, Medicare and Medicaid, the Health Care Financing Administration (HCFA) maintains large data files describing federal health care expenditures, health care providers, and HCFA program beneficiaries [9]. Two quarterly publications, *Health Care Financing Review* (*see* 12.25) and *Health Care Financing Trends* (*see* 12.26) present data on various kinds of national health care expenditures collected by HCFA. These data are the direct result of HCFA's mission to

administer the Medicare and Medicaid programs and related provisions of the Social Security Act and the Public Health Services Act in a manner which: promotes the timely and economic delivery of appropriate quality health care to eligible beneficiaries, promotes beneficiary awareness of the services for which they are eligible and improves the accessibility of those services, and promotes efficiency and quality within the total health care delivery system [10].

HCFA, along with the NCHS, also sponsors the National Medical Care Utilization and Expenditure Survey, included in the *Vital and Health Statistics Series* and designed to obtain data on health insurance coverage, health services use, charges, and sources of payment.

Although the NCHS, CDC, and HCFA are three of the most prolific agencies within the federal government that collect and disseminate statistics, nearly every agency produces statistics of some kind. The National Institutes of Health (NIH), for example, conduct research in the areas of cancer, heart disease, infectious diseases, child health and development, neurological diseases, etc. They can be an important source of statistical information on incidence, prevalence, and cost of treating these conditions. Publications from the NIH are irregular, however, and usually focus on a particular disease. Collecting data is not a major responsibility of the NIH and it is gathered in support of research programs.

Although outside of the Department of Health and Human Services, the Bureau of the Census conducts the decennial census. This national census is the most comprehensive demographic survey in the country and is invaluable for epidemiological research.

The National Technical Information Service (NTIS) of the Department of Commerce also publishes a number of documents of interest to those engaged in health research where statistics are needed. These documents are generally produced on microfiche and are accessed through the *Government Reports & Announcements Index* (*see* 6.3). Recent publications of interest include *Physician's Practice Costs and Incomes Survey, Physicians: Geographic Distribution,* and *Report to the President and Congress on the Status of Health Personnel in the United States.*

International Agencies

The problems of dealing with national statistics are magnified 100-fold when dealing with the difficulties encountered with international statistics. Questions about reliability and comparability must be raised with all statistics, but particularly those produced in developing countries, where efforts are often made to present a better picture of conditions than actually exists and where reporting mechanisms may be slow or ineffectual. In some areas, for example, infant deaths are not counted if the infant is less than six months old, and often persons will die before a complete diagnosis can be made. Organizations such as the United Nations; the Pan American Health Organization; United Nations Educational, Scientific, and Cultural Organization (Unesco), and the International Labor Organization develop useful statistical data incidental to their primary purposes.

The World Health Organization (WHO) serves as the primary international agency in the health field. It conducts extensive programs in the treatment and prevention of diseases, the training of health personnel, and the collection and dissemination of information, including statistics. It assists countries with the development of collecting methods and also publishes the most comprehensive set of international health statistics available in *World Health Statistics Quarterly* (*see* 12.33) and *World Health Statistics Annual* (*see* 12.34). Also of importance in reporting infectious diseases and indigenous health epidemics is the *Weekly Epidemiological Record* (*see* 12.36).

Private Organizations

In addition to governmental agencies, a number of private organizations exist which are prolific producers of statistics. Among these are the professional societies and associations such as the American Medical Association, American Hospital Association, American Dental Association, National League for Nursing, American Nurses Association, and Association of American Medical Colleges. These societies conduct and publish surveys of their membership and their activities or special studies that reveal statistical information unavailable elsewhere. Voluntary and other private organizations such as the American Cancer Society and the Cystic Fibrosis Association can be important sources of statistics in their areas of interest. In fact, almost any association that represents an investment in the health care industry will have a statistical publication of one sort or another.

Publications of important representative organizations are discussed in the "Selected Bibliography of Statistical Sources" section.

SECONDARY SOURCES

Much statistical information remains hidden in journal articles and serial publications. Although journal articles usually present rather specific studies or surveys of a small population, they may be the only sources available for data on a subject. To find statistical information tucked away in journals and serials, secondary sources such as indexes, abstracts, and online databases must be used.

Indexes and Abstracts

The most useful secondary sources are *Index Medicus, American Statistics Index, Index to International Statistics,* and the *Statistical Reference Index.*

Using *Index Medicus,* one can locate the relevant MeSH (Medical Subject Heading) term and then look under the appropriate subheading. Subheadings that identify articles containing statistics are economics, manpower, mortality, epidemiology, supply and distribution, trends, and utilization. For example, statistical information on lung cancer can be found under the MeSH term "LUNG NEOPLASMS" and the subheading "epidemiology" in the July 1991 issue of *Index Medicus* in an article titled "The Prevalence and Age Distribution of Peripheral Pulmonary Hamartomas in Adult Males," in the *South African Medical Journal,* 79(5):247-49: March 2, 1991. For locating more general articles on demography or vital statistics, subject headings such as "DEMOGRAPHY," "VITAL STATISTICS," "MORBIDITY," "MORTALITY," "INFANT MORTALITY," "EPIDEMIOLOGY," or "LIFE EXPECTANCY" can be used.

Of particular interest among the approximately 3,058 journals indexed for *Index Medicus* are the *Vital and Health Statistics Series* of NCHS, *MMWR, World Health Statistics Quarterly,* the *American Journal of Epidemiology, Demography,* and the *WHO Epidemiological Record.*

12.1 *American Statistics Index.* Washington, DC, Congressional Information Service, 1973- . Annual, monthly supplements.

12.2 *International Index of Statistics.* Washington, DC, Congressional Information Service, 1983- . Annual, monthly supplements.

12.3 *Statistical Reference Index.* Washington, DC, Congressional Information Service, 1980- . Annual, monthly supplements.

American Statistics Index (ASI) claims to be the master index to all federal government publications that contain statistical information.

Specifically, the purpose of ASI is to perform the following functions, promptly and comprehensively:

Identify the statistical data published by all branches and agencies of the Federal Government.
Catalog the publications in which these data appear, providing full bibliographic information about each publication.
Announce new publications as they appear.
Describe the contents of the publications fully.
Index this information in full subject detail.
Micropublish virtually all the publications covered by ASI, thereby providing, on a continuing basis, reliable access to the statistics themselves [11].

As such, the *Index* is virtually the only key to ephemeral publications such as *Advance Data* and can be a useful tool in locating information in unexpected places. For periodical literature published by the federal government, *American Statistics Index* gives an open entry for the title followed by analytics of particular issues appearing during the period covered by the index. For all items covered, detailed information is provided about the nature of the data and the parameters they cover. Many points of access are provided, among them subjects, titles, agency report numbers, and such special categories as census division by occupation or age.

The Congressional Information Service began publishing the *International Index of Statistics (IIS)* in 1983. Issued monthly with annual cumulations, this index covers statistical publications of international intergovernmental organizations, including the United Nations, European Communities, Organization for Economic Cooperation and Development (OECD), and approximately forty other organizations. Since 1980, the Congressional Information Service has published the *Statistical Reference Index (SRI)*, yet another monthly index with annual cumulations, which indexes nonfederal U. S. sources including trade, professional, and other nonprofit associations; business organizations; commercial publishers; independent research centers; state government agencies; and university research centers. These three Congressional Information Services indexes are invaluable tools for locating health-related statistics.

An additional index that proves helpful is the *Population Index* published by the Office of Population Research, Princeton University. *Population Index* contains published literature from books and journals primarily on population and related topics such as trends in population growth, mortality, fertility, life expectancy, and socioeconomic characteristics of the population. It is an especially valuable source for information on developing countries. Each issue also lists the official statistical publications of countries throughout the world.

Databases

MEDLINE (*see* 5.1), based on *Index Medicus*, is an efficient way to locate statistical information in journal articles, as is the Health Planning and Administration database (*see* 5.8), which contains citations to journals covered by *Index Medicus, Hospital Literature Index*, and, in a one-time load in May 1983, monographs, monograph chapters, theses, and technical reports submitted from the National Health Planning Information Center. The latter database emphasizes information on health care resources, financing, and other topics related to administration and planning.

POPLINE (*see* 5.11) includes citations from *Population Index* and can be helpful in locating references to articles dealing with population and vital statistics topics. It is currently available from NLM and on CD-ROM from Johns Hopkins University Population Information Program.

ASI, IIS, and *SRI* (*see* 12.1, 12.2, 12.3) are accessible through DIALOG and the CD-ROM product Statistical Masterfile, which is also produced by the Congressional Information Service and allows simultaneous searching of all three indexes. The three indexes can be purchased together, separately, or in any combination in this CD-ROM format which is updated quarterly.

GENERAL STRATEGY FOR LOCATING STATISTICAL INFORMATION

Although the collection and publication of health statistics is not as organized and comprehensive as it could be for ease of access, there is an abundance of reference sources. The question, then, is how to use the available material to its fullest. As with any other area of reference work, a logical approach should be used to find the sought-after statistic.

First, the librarian or information seeker should categorize the question. What is the subject of the request? Into what type of health statistics does it fall—for example, is it a question about vital statistics, chronic or infectious disease, or does it have to do with health manpower, utilization, or economics? Does it deal only with demographic data?

Second, during the reference interview, the researcher should determine the specific variables desired. What is the population (age, sex, race) or geographic area (national, state, city) of interest? How current should the data be, and what time period should they cover?

Once the true nature of the request is determined, the next step is to recall the available primary sources for the data. Who collects this type of data?

Is one agency specifically responsible for regular collection and dissemination of the statistics? How frequent and current is it?

If a particular primary source does not come to mind, the librarian can seek assistance through secondary sources such as the source guides or general compilations of data. This step will sometimes lead to the answer directly or to an appropriate publication or agency. A telephone call to the state or federal agency may yield unpublished data to fulfill the request. If the statistic cannot be located by these means, the librarian can turn to additional secondary sources such as indexes, abstracts, or online databases. Furthermore, the information may be located in a journal article. Those who become familiar with primary sources, and what they contain, should be able to skip to the secondary sources directly when necessary.

When all the known and logical sources have been tapped with no satisfactory results, it may be appropriate to abandon the search or, preferably, to confer with the client to explain the situation and seek reformulation of the request. Briefly, then, the logical steps are

1. Determine the subject of the request.
2. Seek the specifics of the data request from the patron.
3. Consider likely sources of the statistic in the universe of data collection.
4. Consult appropriate primary sources.
5. Search secondary sources if there is no logical primary source.
6. Reformulate the request if no satisfactory data are located.

SELECTED BIBLIOGRAPHY OF STATISTICAL SOURCES

From among the vast number of statistical reference works available in the health care field, a few have been selected and are described here. Criteria for selection are that these works are either major compilations or are representative of a particular subject or type of data that can be accessed. By gaining a general idea of what is available, the reader will be able to deal with reference questions in the area of statistics in a logical and productive fashion.

Source Guides

12.4 Wash, Jim and Boothmer, James A. *Vital and Health Statistics Series: An Annotated Checklist and Index to the Publications of the "Rainbow Series."* Westport, CT, Greenwood Press, 1991.

This work lists, annotates, and indexes all of the reports that have been published in the four series of the U.S. National Health Survey (Series A-D) and the series of the National Center for Health Statistics. The reports are arranged by series, then by report number within the series. Each entry has standard bibliographic information. There is a title index as well as an author and a subject index. The subject index can be useful to zero in on a particular disease or population. Coverage is from reports published from 1958 through March 1991, making it quite current.

12.5 *Catalog of Publications of the National Center for Health Statistics.* Hyattsville, MD, National Center for Health Statistics, 1979- . Formerly: *Current Listing and Topical Index to the Vital and Health Statistics Series,* 1962-1978.

The most recent *Catalog of Publications of the NCHS* covers reports issued 1980-1989 and is periodically supplemented by *Publication Notes.* It provides the simplest way of determining what the NCHS has published recently in each of its series and periodicals as well as other miscellaneous publications. Availability and ordering information are given for each publication. Part I is a listing of its publications, arranged by series and format. Part II is a listing of journal articles by NCHS staff. Part III is an index to health topics.

12.6 Weise, Frieda. *Health Statistics: A Guide to Information Sources.* Health Affairs Information Guide Series, vol. 4. Detroit, MI, Gale, 1980.

Health Statistics is a guide to basic sources of vital and health statistics in the United States. The annotated bibliography provides details on the coverage, completeness, and uniformity of statistics reported by local, state, and federal governments as well as by private health organizations and professional associations. This information, presented in an organized format, will aid the often difficult search for health data. Although published in 1980, this source provides a useful compendium of publications, many of which are in continuing series, and is very useful as a starting point for much statistical research in health-related fields. A new edition is planned for publication in 1995.

Included within the scope of *Health Statistics* are data on natality and mortality, marriage and divorce, morbidity, health care facilities, health manpower, health services utilization, health care costs and expenditures, education of health professionals, and population characteristics. Following the main bibliography of sources of vital and health statistics are file appendices covering additional sources of information. Separate appendices are devoted to newsletters and journals, government agencies, associations, regional depository libraries, and suppliers of bibliographic data files.

Compilations

12.7 Bureau of the Census. *Statistical Abstract of the United States*. Washington, DC, U.S. Government Printing Office, 1878- . Annual.

The *Statistical Abstract* is one of the first places to look when answering any statistical question, not just those related to health care. This single-volume work contains more than 1,400 statistical tables and charts that address the nation's social organization, economy, and politics, as well as the nation's health. The *Statistical Abstract* contains information on everything from population density to the average price per pound of the catch of U.S. fisheries. It is an indispensable reference tool for any library.

The major strength of the *Statistical Abstract* lies in the fact that it serves as a primary and secondary source for a wide range of national statistical data. It essentially consists of excerpts, summaries, or compilations of data gathered and published in greater detail elsewhere. The original publications, both governmental and private, are always cited and can be referred to if more specificity is required.

Although the *Statistical Abstract* is published yearly, the data contained within are usually presented in multiyear groupings. There is, however, no guarantee on the currency of data or consistency of presentation from table to table, graph to graph, etc. In the 1990 edition, for example, some of the figures presented are as recent as 1990, but in other cases the most recent data may be a much as three years old. Furthermore, the data, although extensive, are not always presented on a state-by-state basis, and regional subdivisions are only occasionally provided.

The basic organization of the *Statistical Abstract* has remained fairly consistent over the years: broad subject sections, appendices, and a strong index emphasizing the subject approach. Each section, in turn, contains an explanatory preface that clearly defines major terms, concepts, and issues. Beginning with the 1977 edition, as a reflection of the times, more health-related data are being included in two sections, "Vital Statistics" and "Health and Nutrition." Additional relevant material is contained in the sections on "Population," "Social Insurance and Human Services," "Banking, Finance, and Insurance," "Science," and "Comparative International Statistics."

The appendices of the *Statistical Abstract* contain, among other things, a complete current listing of population data for the official Standard Metropolitan Statistical Areas (SMSA), a guide to sources of statistics, guides to state and foreign statistical abstracts, and the "Index to Tables Having Historical Statistics, Colonial Times to 1970 Series."

12.8 Bureau of the Census. *Historical Statistics of the United States: Colonial Times to 1970.* Bicentennial ed. Washington, DC, U.S. Government Printing Office, 1975.

Historical Statistics explicitly serves as a companion piece to the *Statistical Abstract.* The scope of coverage is identical, the mode of presentation is similar, and its usefulness as both a primary and secondary source endows it with equal importance. The publication pattern, however, differs, there having been only two previous editions (1949 and 1960).

Historical Statistics is organized by broad subject chapters similar, though not identical, to those of the *Statistical Abstract,* and by "time series." A time series refers to a single vertical column of data, each increment of which extends the data backwards over time. A table of data, in turn, consists of several time series grouped together. The time period index correlates the chapter headings with twenty-year periods in U.S. history and uses the time series, rather than page numbers, as points of reference. Furthermore, the appendix in the *Statistical Abstract,* "Index to Tables Having Historical Statistics, Colonial Times to 1970 Series," correlates appropriate time series in the current volume. Therefore, by noting the time series, one can easily turn to the *Statistical Abstract* for more current data. However, no provision was made for such ease of movement from the more recent data to the historical. Two of the most valuable chapters for health statistics are "Population" and "Vital Statistics and Health and Medical Care." Both chapters contain series of tables (for example, Series B 107-115, Expectation of Life [in years] at Birth, by Race and Sex 1900-1970).

Each series contains a preface that provides a discussion of the type of data in the tables, principles of data collection, primary sources of data, and problems associated with interpretation of the data. This preface information is extremely important as it impacts on the possible uses of the data. It also contains probably the most definitive information on primary sources available.

Historical Statistics is rich in information. Like the *Statistical Abstract,* it is an appropriate starting point in answering any statistical question with an historical emphasis.

12.9 National Center for Health Statistics. *Health: United States.* Washington, DC, U. S. Government Printing Office, 1975/76- . Annual.

Health: United States is an annual report on the health status of the nation, submitted by the secretary of Health and Human Services to the President and Congress in compliance with Section 308 of the Public Health Service Act. The report generally consists of two parts, the first being a thorough presentation of an important topic that changes from year to year. The second part consists of detailed statistical tables that are organized around major subject areas—health status and determinants, utilization of health resources, health care resources, and health care expenditures. The appendices provide descriptions and limitations of the data sources and a glossary of terms, each of which is extremely valuable in itself. Since 1980, every third year *Health: United States* includes a section titled "Prevention Profile." This section "assembles the most recent data available for areas in which preventive actions are now being taken and/or in which opportunities for new activities have been well charted" [12]. The 134 detailed tables from the 1990 edition are available on disc from the Government Printing Office and are especially useful for persons engaged in flow sheets and LOTUS software manipulations. No reference librarian should be without *Health: United States* because it contains the most recently available published or unpublished summary data on the topics covered.

Vital and Morbidity Statistics

12.10 National Center for Health Statistics. *Vital Statistics of the United States.* Washington, DC, U. S. Government Printing Office, 1937- . Vol. 1: *Natality;* Vol. 2: *Mortality;* Vol. 3: *Marriage and Divorce.*

Although perpetually out of date by at least five years, *Vital Statistics of the United States* nevertheless comprises the final word on births, deaths, fetal deaths, marriages, and divorces in the United States. The series is issued yearly, but multiyear trends are often contained in extensive and often surprisingly geographic detail, occasionally down to the township level. The presence of other demographic parameters such as race, sex, and age encourages consultation of the volumes for questions that initially appear to be either too local or too particular in scope for inclusion in a "national" series. For example, such esoteric information as "Live Births by Age of Mother, Live Birth Order, and Race" can be found for a particular state without having to locate that state's separately published vital statistics.

The series contains no index. A highly detailed table of contents can provide adequate access if the user has already gained some familiarity with the work. In addition, volume 1 contains a chart, "General Pattern of Vital Registration and Statistics in the United States," which illustrates the process by which a birth, death, marriage, or divorce actually enters the reporting system. A technical appendix to each volume provides historical information, definitions, forms, and tables that further explain the means by which statistics are produced.

12.11 *Monthly Vital Statistics Report; Provisional Statistics from the National Center for Health Statistics.* Hyattsville, MD, National Center for Health Statistics, 1952-

Monthly Vital Statistics Report (MVSR) is a preview of the data that will appear later in *Vital Statistics of the United States.* Each issue covers one month, providing figures on live births, deaths, natural increase in the population, marriages, divorces, and infant deaths. Multiyear trends are charted, and comparative statistics are given for the month covered in previous years as well as twelve-month cumulations. Each issue also contains state and regional statistics; age, race, and sex breakdowns on death rates; and, like the *Vital Statistics of the United States,* uses *The International Classification of Diseases* (see 9.16) for cause of death. *MVSR* gives numbers and rates for seventy-two selected causes of death. However, the data in *MVSR* are provisional; the detail for which *Vital Statistics of the United States* is noted is absent from the smaller publication. Most of the data in *MVSR* are based on samples rather than on whole populations and, therefore, are subject to error.

In addition to regular monthly issues, *MVSR* also presents "final data" in supplementary issues. These reports represent summary tabulations of annual vital statistics data. For example, "Advance Report of Final Marriage Statistics, 1988" was published as a supplement to volume 40 of *Monthly Vital Statistics Report,* thus providing current data well in advance of the comprehensive data that will appear in volume 3—*Marriage and Divorce, Vital Statistics of the United States*—which will probably not be available until 1994.

The strengths of this newsletter certainly more than compensate for its weaknesses. It is current and constant. Data provided are usually for the third month preceding month of issue. Because it carries the same type of information from month to month, one quickly learns what to expect from it. *Monthly Vital Statistics Report* belies its humble exterior and should find regular use in those collections for which demographic information and vital statistics are in demand.

12.12 *Vital and Health Statistics Series.* Hyattsville, MD, National Center for Health Statistics, 1963- .

Also known as the "Rainbow Series," the *Vital and Health Statistics Series* exemplifies one of the great paradoxes of statistical reference: data contained in it represent the National Center for Health Statistics at its best; however, access to the data shows the Center at its worst. The *Vital and Health Statistics Series* actually consists of eighteen irregularly issued subseries of data compiled through the surveys and studies of the NCHS. The data are presented along with samples of the questionnaires, technical definitions, etc. Everything from "Serum Lipids and Lipoproteins of Hispanics, 1982-84" to "Birth and Fertility Rates by Education: 1980 and 1985" can be found.

Unfortunately, pinpointing the data is rather difficult. Indexing these publications in detail is quite impossible; therefore, the most likely title must be chosen, followed by browsing through the issue. However, help is offered through the *Vital and Health Statistics Series: An Annotated Checklist and Index to the Publications of the "Rainbow Series"* (*see* 12.4) as well as by *American Statistics Index* (*see* 12.1). Because the series is covered in *Index Medicus*, it may turn up in a search of the *Index* or MEDLINE database as well.

In spite of these difficulties, the "Rainbow Series" is a must for reference librarians. Series 10 and Series 11, covering the National Health Interview Survey and the National Health Examination Survey, are particularly important because they contain prevalence data on chronic diseases collected by NCHS and unavailable elsewhere on a national scale. The various active subseries and the areas they cover are listed in Table 12-2 [13].

12.13 *Advance Data from Vital and Health Statistics of the National Center for Health Statistics.* Hyattsville, MD, National Center for Health Statistics, 1976- .

The full title to *Advance Data,* provided in the above citation, accurately describes this short (five to twenty pages), irregularly issued newsletter: a vehicle by which information from the various surveys conducted by the National Center for Health Statistics gains early release to the public. Most of the information contained in *Advance Data* will eventually find its way into the *Vital and Health Statistics Series.* Each issue addresses one topic, ranging from "Use of Vitamin and Mineral Supplements in the United States: Current Users, Types of Products, and Nutrients," to "Children's Exposure to Environmental Cigarette Smoke Before and After Birth," and is replete with the necessary charts and tables, footnotes, cross-references, definitions, forms, and technical notes.

Advance Data, however, suffers acutely from the weakness of the other government-issued statistical series. The wealth of information often remains a hidden treasure due to lack of subject access. It is a publication that must be monitored to be used effectively; however, it is covered in *American Statistics Index, Energy Information Abstracts, Environment Abstracts, Excerpta Medica, Hospital Literature Index,* and *Population Index,* and is searchable online in the Health Planning and Administration database. The various NCHS catalogs (*see* 12.5) offer a complete listing of the titles issued thus

Table 12-2. Vital and Health Statistics Series

Series 1. *Programs and Collection Procedures.* Reports describing the general programs of the National Center for Health Statistics and its offices and divisions and the data collection methods used. They also include definitions and other material necessary for understanding the data.

Series 2. *Data Evaluation and Methods Research.* Studies of new statistical methodology, including experimental tests of new survey methods, studies of vital statistics collection methods, new analytical techniques, objective evaluations of reliability of collected data, and contributions to statistical theory. Studies also include comparison of U. S. methodology with those of other countries.

Series 3. *Analytical and Epidemiological Studies.* Reports presenting analytical or interpretive studies based on vital and health statistics, carrying the analysis further than the expository types of reports in the other series.

Series 4. *Documents and Committee Reports.* Final reports of major committees concerned with vital and health statistics and documents such as recommended model vital registration laws and revised birth and death certificates.

Series 5. *Comparative International Vital and Health Statistics Reports.* Analytical and descriptive reports comparing U.S. vital and health statistics with those of other countries.

Series 6. *Cognition and Survey Measurement.* Reports from the National Laboratory for Collaborative Research in Cognition and Survey Measurement using methods of cognitive science to design, evaluate, and test survey instruments.

Series 10. *Data From the National Health Interview Survey.* Statistics on illness; accidental injuries; disability; use of hospital, medical, dental, and other services; and other health-related topics—all based on data collected in the continuing national household interview survey.

Series 11. *Data From the National Health Examination Survey and the National Health and Nutrition Examination Survey.* Data from direct examination, testing, and measurement of national samples of the civilian noninstitutionalized population provide the basis for (1) estimates of the medically defined prevalence of specific diseases in the United States and the distributions of

Table 12-2 (continued)

the population with respect to physical, physiological, and psychological characteristics; and (2) analysis of relationships among the various measurements without reference to an explicit finite universe of persons.

Series 12.   *Data From the Institutionalized Population Survey.* Discontinued in 1975. Reports from these surveys are included in Series 13.

Series 13.   *Data on Health Resources Utilization.* Statistics on the utilization of health manpower and facilities providing long-term care, ambulatory care, hospital care, and family planning services.

Series 14.   *Data on Health Resources: Manpower and Facilities.* Statistics on the numbers, geographic distribution, and characteristics of health resources including physicians, dentists, nurses, other health occupations, hospitals, nursing homes, and out-patient facilities.

Series 15.   *Data From Special Surveys.* Statistics on health and health-related topics collected in special surveys that are not a part of the continuing data systems of the National Center for Health Statistics.

Series 16.   *Compilations of Advance Data From Vital and Health Statistics.* These reports provide early release of data from the National Center for Health Statistics' health and demographic surveys. Many of these releases are followed by detailed reports in the *Vital and Health Statistics Series.*

Series 20.   *Data on Mortality.* Various statistics on mortality other than as included in regular annual or monthly reports. Special analyses by cause of death, age, and other demographic variables; geographic and time series analyses; and statistics on characteristics of death not available from the vital records based on sample surveys of those records.

Series 21.   *Data on Natality, Marriage, and Divorce.* Various statistics on natality, marriage, and divorce other than as included in regular annual or monthly reports. Special analyses by demographic variables; geographic and time series analyses; studies of fertility; and statistics on characteristics of births not available from the vital records based on sample surveys of those records.

Table 12-2 (continued)

Series 22.	*Data From the National Mortality and Natality Surveys.* Discontinued in 1975. Reports from these sample surveys based on vital records are included in Series 20 and 21, respectively.
Series 23.	*Data From the National Survey of Family Growth.* Statistics on fertility, family formation and dissolution, family planning, and related maternal and infant health topics derived from a periodic survey of a nationwide probability sample of women fifteen to forty-four years of age.
Series 24.	*Compilations of Data on Natality, Mortality, Marriage, Divorce, and Induced Terminations of Pregnancy.* Advance reports of births, deaths, marriages, and divorces are based on final data from the National Vital Statistics System and are published annually as supplements to the *Monthly Vital Statistics Report* (*MVSR*). These reports are followed by the publication of detailed data in *Vital Statistics of the United States* annual volumes. Other reports including induced terminations of pregnancy, issued periodically as supplements to the *MVSR*, provide selected findings based on data from the National Vital Statistics System and may be followed by detailed reports in *Vital and Health Statistics Series.*

far, and can be used as a quick reference to see if a particular subject has been covered in the series.

12.14 *MMWR: Morbidity and Mortality Weekly Report.* Atlanta, GA, Centers for Disease Control, 1952- .

12.15 *Annual Summary MMWR: Morbidity and Mortality Weekly Report.* Atlanta, GA, Centers for Disease Control, 1952- .

12.16 *Surveillance Summaries MMWR: Morbidity and Mortality Weekly Report.* Atlanta, GA, Centers for Disease Control, 1983- . Quarterly.

12.17 *Recommendations and Reports: Morbidity and Mortality Weekly Report.* Atlanta, GA, Centers for Disease Control, 1989- .

The Centers for Disease Control have begun referring to their publications collectively as the *Morbidity and Mortality Information Series (MMIS).* Although this title does not appear on any of the title pages, the above publications fall into this series.

At the heart of *MMWR* are currently three statistical tables: (1) cases of specified notifiable diseases, United States (cumulative for the year); (2) cases of selected notifiable diseases, United States (cumulative for current year and previous year); and (3) deaths for all causes in 121 U.S. cities (cumulative for current year). These tables provide the user with extremely current data on the occurrence of various diseases in the country.

Each issue also contains three to five special sections: "Epidemiologic Notes and Reports," "Current Trends," "Effectiveness in Disease and Injury Prevention," "Notice to Readers," and "International Notes." These special sections and their topics vary from week to week, but they provide larger pictures of items of national and international interest. "Current Trends," for example, might have an update on acquired immunodeficiency syndrome (AIDS) or on childhood cancers.

The *Annual Summary* is published as the last issue in each volume of *MMWR* and covers the previous year. That is, the 1989 *Annual Summary* appeared as volume 38, number 54, in 1990. This issue does not, however, supersede the special reports in the previous weekly issues, which should be retained. This statistical summary contains summarized morbidity and mortality data for each of the forty-nine currently reportable conditions and data on nonnotifiable conditions from the surveillance programs, thus providing information on the nation's health unavailable elsewhere. The *Annual Index* issue is published as the 53rd issue in each volume of *MMWR* and covers the previous year. That is, the 1989 *Annual Index* appeared as volume 38, number 53, in 1990. Supplements, surveillance summaries, and weekly issues of the *MMWR* are included in this index. In addition to complete subject coverage of *MMWR*, it also lists *MMWR* publications other than the weekly issues that are considered part of the volume. As such, it is an important tool for bibliographic control and subject access to the *MMWR* publications.

MMWR is indexed by the *American Statistics Index* and is covered by *Index Medicus* and MEDLINE. Full text is available on BRS, DIALOG, and through the Internet from NIH.

Surveillance Summaries has absorbed the previously irregular series of *Surveillance Reports* into one report. Published quarterly, the *Summaries* normally contain annual data on a number of conditions monitored in the surveillance programs of the CDC. Conditions such as ectopic pregnancy, Rocky Mountain spotted fever, and pneumoconiosis in coal miners are among the more than twenty monitored conditions. The *MMWR Annual Summary* complements the quarterly publication in its coverage of surveillance data. *Recommendations and Reports* is a relatively recent addition to the *MMWR* and includes recommendations and guidelines on the prevention of infectious diseases, new ICD-9-CM codes for infectious diseases, and

Public Health Service reports on health benefits and risks of various treatments.

Health Resources and Utilization

12.18 National Center for Health Statistics. *Health Resources Statistics.* 1976-77 ed. Washington, DC, U. S. Government Printing Office, 1979.

Health Resources Statistics is probably too out-of-date to be useful for primary information; however, more recent data on the topics available in this source may be obtained by consulting the agency originally responsible for the data. *Health Resources Statistics* is a summary of data regarding health manpower, facilities, and services compiled by the Division of Health Manpower and Facilities Statistics of the National Center for Health Statistics, and as such is a useful tool for locating who might currently be publishing data, as well as for sources of historical data.

Facilities

12.19 *Hospital Statistics.* Chicago, American Hospital Association, 1972- . Annual.

12.20 *Length of Stay by Diagnosis and Operation.* Ann Arbor, MI, Healthcare Knowledge Resources, 1986- . Annual. Formed by the union of: *Length of Stay by Diagnosis* and *Length of Stay by Operation.* Ann Arbor, MI, Commission on Professional and Hospital Activities.

Data on health facilities and utilization may be found in several sources. The *Vital and Health Statistics Series 13* and *Series 14*—"Data on Health Resources Utilization" and "Data on Health Resources" respectively—offer data on various types of facilities and their utilization, including hospitals, nursing homes, and family planning services. *Hospital Statistics,* however, is a more current source used by hospitals themselves. It contains information collected by the American Hospital Association in its annual survey of hospitals. A short introduction defines terms used and discusses characteristics and trends in hospital utilization. It also includes tables on hospital capacity, utilization, personnel, finances, facilities, and services, with trends from 1946 to date. It includes data by census division, state, SMSA, 100 largest central cities, and outlying territories, cross-tabulated variously by hospital bed-size group, control, and service classifications. *Hospital Statistics* is the source to use for answers to such questions as "What percentage of hospitals in Mississippi have speech pathology services?" or "How many hospital beds are there in Elmira, New York?"

Length of Stay by Diagnosis and Operation offers another type of data: statistical tables that describe hospital stay for the year. Published in multiple volumes covering the United States, the four census regions, and Canada, the data are intended to "provide a valuable perspective for utilization review, quality assurance professionals, physicians, consultants, hospital administrators, third party payors, and researchers interested in cost containment and quality care" (1989 ed., *United States* volume, Introduction, v). Using the tables, one can determine such statistics as what the average length of hospital stay is for cases of acute appendicitis with peritonitis if the patient is twenty years old. Also included in this series are *Pediatric Length of Stay by Diagnosis and Operation, United States; Geriatric Length of Stay by Diagnosis and Operation, United States; Psychiatric Length of Stay;* and *Length of Stay by DRG and Payment Source.*

Manpower

> 12.21 *Physician Characteristics and Distribution in the U.S.* Chicago, American Medical Association, 1981- . Annual.
>
> 12.22 *U.S. Medical Licensure Statistics and Current Licensure Requirements 1990-* . Chicago, American Medical Association. Annual. Formed from: *Medical Licensure Statistics 1971-* and *U.S. Medical Licensure Statistics 1980-81—and Licensure Requirements 1982-* . Title varies: *Medical Licensure Statistics, Licensure Requirements, U.S. Medical Licensure Statistics...and Licensure Requirements.*

These two AMA publications were previously included in one volume entitled *Physician Distribution and Medical Licensure in the U.S. (1974-80).* Together, they contain the most comprehensive set of physician manpower statistics available. *Physician Characteristics* provides extensive data on the number of physicians by major professional activity and specialty for the nation, census region, state, county, and metropolitan area, as well as separate summary tabulations for women and foreign medical graduates. Physician population characteristics such as age, sex, board certification, year of graduation, and country of origin are also given, along with trend data highlighting physician characteristics and distribution.

Types of questions that may be answered by this work are "How many physicians are there in Laramie, Wyoming?" and "How many board certified physicians are there in neurology?" The most recent edition does not include any socioeconomic data for the population in the geographic areas covered, nor does it include economic data for physicians. This data is covered in *Socioeconomic Characteristics of Medical Practice* (*see* 12.28) and *Physician Marketplace Statistics* (*see* 12.29).

Licensure Statistics provides data on the number of licenses issued by state medical boards, examination activity of the National Board of Medical Examiners, number of physicians awarded National Board Certificates by

Medical School, and also contains extensive licensure policies of state medical licensing boards and current board standards for administration of the FLEX examination.

12.23 *Facts About Nursing.* Kansas City, MO, American Nurses Association, 1935- . Biannual.

Facts About Nursing can be relied upon to supply almost any data need related to nursing manpower, distribution, or education. Chapters are devoted to the distribution of registered nurses, nursing education, economic status of registered nurses, allied nursing personnel, and related vital and health statistics information. Each chapter comprises several sections containing many tables, and each section has an illuminating introductory discussion of the data-gathering activities and analysis of the data presented in the tables. Recent editions have expanded the help wanted advertising index, including information on advanced specialized practice and present licensure requirements. *Facts About Nursing* is an indispensable tool for those in the nursing profession and for health sciences librarians.

Education

12.24 *Medical Education in the United States. Annual Report.* Chicago, American Medical Association, 1901- .

The tradition of devoting an entire issue of the *Journal of the American Medical Association (JAMA)* to medical education began in 1901. The "education issue," as it is called, currently provides information on undergraduate medical education, U. S. medical school finances, graduate medical education in the United States, continuing medical education, allied health education and accreditation, and medical education programs sponsored by government agencies. It also includes membership of committees on education and a list of medical schools in the United States and Canada.

The questions that could be answered by consulting the *Annual Report* include, "What percentage of students enrolled in medical school are Hispanic?" and "How many residency programs are there in pediatrics?" Extensive text accompanies tables; several appendices provide further detailed data for individual schools. The *Annual Report* will fill most needs for statistics on the education of physicians and on medical schools, but data on the education of the allied health professionals must be obtained from their respective professional associations. Examples of publications from other professional societies are the American Dental Association's *Annual Report on Dental Education,* the National League for Nursing's annually published *NLN Nursing Data Book,* and the American Nurses Association's *Facts About Nursing (see* 12.23).

Health Care Costs and Expenditures

12.25 U.S. Health Care Financing Administration. *Health Care Financing Review.* Vol. 1- , 1979- . Quarterly.

12.26 U.S. Health Care Financing Administration. *Health Care Financing Trends.* Vol. 1- , 1979- . Quarterly.

12.27 *Source Book of Health Insurance Data.* Washington, DC, Health Insurance Association of America, 1959- . Annual.

The Health Care Financing Administration (HCFA) has the federal responsibility for publishing health care financing data. Both HCFA publications are published quarterly and present similar data. In the *Review,* the annually published summary tables on national health expenditures (formerly in the *Social Security Bulletin)* can be located. These annual summaries cover total amounts, sources of money, and expenditures. For example, the tables show the percentage of hospital care costs paid by Medicare funds and the per capita expenditures for health care for the year. Data also show trends over several years. *Health Care Financing Trends* presents quarterly data and analyses on national health expenditures, community hospital statistics, consumer price indexes, employment hours, earnings of health workers, and related information.

Although these two publications cover the topic quite thoroughly, the *Source Book of Health Insurance Data* contains supplementary financial information. It is a report of the private health insurance business in the United States and provides details on the major forms of health insurance: hospital, surgical, physician's expense, major medical, disability, and dental. Summary data on health care costs and health resources are included. One of the more interesting tables in the 1990 *Source Book* is "Cost of Having a Baby."

Publications from both the federal and the private sector should be kept in mind when searching for financial data because each presents information from a different viewpoint.

12.28 *Socioeconomic Characteristics of Medical Practice.* Chicago, American Medical Association, 1983- . Annual.

12.29 *Physician Marketplace Statistics.* Chicago, American Medical Association, 1988- . Annual.

Socioeconomic Characteristics of Medical Practice contains information on physicians' earnings; medical professional liability claims and premiums;

physicians' practice costs, trends and variations; weeks and hours of practice; use of physician services fees for physician visits; professional expenses of physicians; and physician net income after expenses before taxes. Appendices include extensive information on the design and methodology of the data-gathering techniques used, the socioeconomic monitoring system questionnaire summary, and definitions of variables.

The *Physician Marketplace Statistics* expands the *Socioeconomic Characteristics of Medical Practice* by "providing more detailed breakdowns of Socioeconomic Monitoring System (SMS) information." (Foreword, 1990 edition, iii). As such, it includes SMS information for selected internal medicine and surgical subspecialties, the ten largest states, and selected physician practice arrangements. Fees for selected procedures, measures of Medicare use, and deferred physician compensation statistics are also included. Both books, although quite expensive, are useful reference tools in bringing together detailed statistics on the socioeconomic characteristics of health care, medical practice, and physicians.

Demographic Sources

The decennial *Census of Population* provides the most comprehensive data on demographic and socioeconomic characteristics of the U. S. population. It is important for the health sciences librarian to take the census publications into account, because much research today involves looking at the nation's health in the light of social and economic forces. Additionally, all of the important "rates" (for example, prevalence rate or mortality rate) are based on current population figures. The following are the most important sources of the 1990 census.

12.30 Bureau of Census. *Census Catalog and Guide, 1991.* Washington, DC, U. S. Government Printing Office, 1991.

12.31 Bureau of Census. *1990 Census of Population and Housing.* Washington, DC, U. S. Government Printing Office.

12.32 Bureau of Census. *Current Population Reports.* Washington, DC, U. S. Government Printing Office, 1947- .

The Census Bureau publishes an extensive and impressive amount of data in a variety of different series of publications. To gain an understanding of and appreciation for them, it is extremely valuable to refer to the *Census Catalog and Guide.* Because some data are collected from the entire population and other data from a sample only, one must be aware of the type of data in a given publication. The *Guide* offers a thorough discussion of the data subjects and explains how to locate data for a particular geographic area.

With the 1990 Census, the arrangement of the volumes has changed. The *Census of Population and Housing* volumes present demographic, social, and economic characteristics data on the population. Following is a breakdown of the important population sections of the Census [14].

Summary Population and Housing Characteristics: (CPH-1-nos.) provides population and housing unit costs and statistics on age, sex, race, household relationship, and housing structure for states, local governmental units, other county subdivisions, and American Indian and Alaska Native areas.

General Population Characteristics: (CP-1-nos.) presents detailed statistics on age, sex, race, Hispanic origin, marital status, and household relationship characteristics for states, counties, places of 1,000 or more inhabitants, MCDs (Minor Civil Division) of 1,000 or more inhabitants in selected states, state parts of American Indian and Alaska Native areas, and summary geographic areas.

Social and Economic Characteristics: (CP-2-nos.) focuses on the population subjects collected on a sample basis in 1990. Data will be shown for states, counties, places of 2,500 or more inhabitants, MCDs of 2,500 or more inhabitants in selected states, and the state portion of American Indian and Alaska Native areas.

The Census Bureau also conducts national and regional surveys periodically, aside from the decennial census. The results of these surveys, published in *Current Population Reports,* are issued in the following series.

Series P-20, *Population Characteristics,* contains reports dealing with topics such as fertility and morbidity, usually at the national level.

Series P-23, *Special Studies,* comprises several reports issued each year on such subjects as aging, women, and institutionalized persons.

Series P-25, *Population Estimates and Projections,* includes monthly and annual estimates and projections, such as by age, race, and sex for the United States, the states, or other geographic areas.

A very helpful "Subject Index to Current Population Reports" has been published as No. 144 in the *Special Studies Series,* P-23. It provides handy access to reports dealing with subjects such as elderly, fertility, educational attainment, and poverty data. The reports in the *Special Studies Series,* P-23, are quite comprehensive and include more than census data.

International Sources

12.33 *World Health Statistics Quarterly*. Geneva, Switzerland, World Health Organization, 1978- . Formerly: *Epidemiological and Vital Statistics Report*, 1947-1967; *World Health Statistics Report*, 1968-1977.
12.34 *World Health Statistics Annual*. Geneva, Switzerland, World Health Organization, 1939- .

Both *World Health Statistics Quarterly* and *Annual* are published by the World Health Organization (WHO) and attempt to give a picture of health and vital statistics on a worldwide basis. A cautionary note: the statistical expressions are only as good as the reporting system in each country, and these vary widely in consistency and reliability. Giving some recognition to this problem, WHO has set up an information service on world health statistics, which, among other things, aims to improve the quality and timeliness of information available and to define the limiting factors caused by comparing data generated from many different sources.

The *World Health Statistics Quarterly* has changed character over its years of publication. In 1974, it was reoriented from merely the presentation of data on vital and health statistics to the interpretation of data. It now contains articles that provide data analysis on major health topics, and the current data part of the journal has been curtailed. Recent issues have covered such important worldwide issues as progress in leprosy control, environmental epidemiology, and lifestyles and health. This important journal is indexed in the print and online versions of *Biological Abstracts, Population Index,* and *Index Medicus,* thus making its information quite accessible.

World Health Statistics Annual contains final and "official" (i.e., given to WHO by the competent authorities of the countries concerned) vital statistics, morbidity statistics for the infectious diseases, and information on health resources, usually published several years after the fact. The *Annual* contains a tradition of reporting this information first begun by the League of Nations with its *Annual Epidemiological Report* for 1921-1938 and then taken up by WHO in the *Annual Epidemiological and Vital Statistics* for 1939-1946.

The *Annual* was published in three volumes until 1983. It is now one volume and comprises the following sections: global overview, special topic, vital statistics and life tables, and cause of death. The *Annual* remains the only source that attempts to cover all countries of the world and is a valuable reference tool.

12.35 *Demographic Yearbook*. New York, United Nations Statistical Office, 1948- .

Published by the United Nations, the *Yearbook* presents official demographic statistics for about 220 countries or areas of the world. Generally, it contains basic tables that are published annually, followed by a special topic. The basic tables show world summary population estimates, infant and maternal mortality, general mortality, marriage (here called nuptiality), and divorce. The 1989 issue devoted its special topic to international migration statistics, presenting data on all related matters including, for example, native and foreign-born population by age, sex, and urban or rural residence: each census, 1980-1988. It also includes a detailed section entitled "Technical Notes on the Statistical Tables" to assist readers.

12.36 *Weekly Epidemiological Record.* Geneva, Switzerland, World Health Organization, 1925- .

Published by the World Health Organization, the *Weekly Epidemiological Record* reports on infectious diseases worldwide. Presented in a dual-language format (French and English), it offers continuing reports on the plague, cholera, yellow fever, influenza, AIDS, and other infectious diseases. It is also a useful source for articles on these subjects, as well as reporting international health regulations. Although somewhat haphazard in its statistical coverage, the annual index, published at the end of the year, provides extensive coverage to the weekly issues and is invaluable for locating statistics.

REFERENCES

1. U.S. Department of Commerce, Office of Federal Statistical Policy and Standards. A framework for planning U.S. federal statistics for the 1980s. Washington, DC: U.S. Government Printing Office, 1978:116-17.

2. U.S. Congress, House Committee on Interstate and Foreign Commerce, Subcommittee on Health and Environment. Discursive dictionary of health care. Washington, DC: U.S. Government Printing Office, 1976.

3. Last JM. A dictionary of epidemiology. Edited for the International Epidemiological Association, New York: Oxford University Press, 1983. (second edition published in 1988).

4. Last, JM, ed. Maxcy-Rosenau public health and preventive medicine. 11th ed. New York: Appleton-Century-Crofts, 1980:14.

5. National Office of Vital Statistics. History of organization of the vital statistics system: vital statistics of the United States. V. 1. Washington, DC: U.S. Government Printing Office, 1950:2-19.

6. Vital and health statistics program and collection procedures: origin, program, and operation of the U.S. national health survey. Washington, DC: U.S. Government Printing Office, 1963:15 (Vital and Health Statistics Series, No. 1000-Series 1-No. 1) (Public Health Service Publication).

7. 1987/88 United States government manual. Washington, DC: U.S. Government Printing Office, 1987:298.

8. 1990/91 United States government manual. Washington, DC: U.S. Government Printing Office, 1990:306.

9. U.S. Department of Health, Education, and Welfare. Health statistics plan 1979-80. Washington, DC: U.S. Government Printing Office, 1980:15.

10. Federal Register. Washington, DC: U.S. Government Printing Office, V. 55, No. 49 (March 13, 1990):9363.

11. American Statistics Index. Washington, DC: Congressional Information Service, 1990:vii.

12. Health: United States, 1980. Washington, DC: U.S. Government Printing Office, 1981:267.

13. Series information can be located on the inside back cover of each issue in each series.

14. Census catalog and guide, 1991. Washington, DC: U.S. Government Printing Office, 1991:166-67.

CHAPTER 13

Directories and Biographical Sources

Jo Anne Boorkman

Directories are among the most frequently consulted reference tools. Therefore, one of the major factors to consider when dealing with them is currency. The *Federal Executive Telephone Directory*, for example, is updated every two months to reflect the continuous changes in government. This is probably an extreme example; nevertheless, the accuracy of the information a librarian is able to provide will be related to the timeliness of the directories in the collection. The currency of a directory is often of major importance; when giving a client directory information, it is a good idea to note source and date.

Format is another factor to consider in selecting and using directories. In a reference situation, the client is often in a hurry, so the librarian needs to locate the answer as quickly as possible. It can be frustrating to flip through a directory hoping to find the needed section or to hunt for an index buried in the middle of a volume. Some directories have a convenient alphabetical arrangement. Others frequently are arranged in a geographic or a classified subject format. Directories without indexes can be tedious to use, especially if the requester does not have sufficient information to allow for alternate search strategies. It is imperative that a librarian know the directories in the reference collection.

Some directories are available online from database vendors or on portable files, e.g., disks or CD-ROMs. The electronic formats are sometimes updated more frequently than the print format directories. The frequency of need to access information in a particular directory will often dictate the choice of format for a library. For directories that are accessed infrequently, it may be more cost effective to access the information from a vendor rather than subscribe to the directory. Health sciences librarians have found that frequently used directories are best accessed from the print format rather than disk or CD-ROM. Frequently used directories need the ready access and quick look-up availability that only a book provides. Having the directory available only on disk or CD-ROM may make it immediately unavailable when the equipment needed for its use is tied up by clientele using the machine for database searching. Networked formats (tapes or CD-ROMs on a local area network) are available for some directories; however, licensing costs need to be taken into consideration when considering these formats for a library's collection. A busy reference service may thus find the print format of most directories to be the best value for its collection, with online access to a vendor's database for the most up-to-date information.

BIOGRAPHICAL SOURCES AND DIRECTORIES OF SCIENTISTS

Some of the most frequent reference requests are for biographical or address information. A client wants to know the educational background of a physician before making an appointment, or an insurance company needs to confirm the address of a physician. These questions often appear to be very straightforward and uncomplicated. However, the client does not always know the first name of Dr. Smith in Los Angeles, and Dr. Smith's specialty may be internal medicine, but then again it may be gastroenterology. The insurance secretary just has the doctor's signature, and it "looks like" T. J. Crandell, or is that F. J. Granville? Thus, two seemingly direct requests for information are often less than clear. With biographical questions, it is important to find out as much information from the client as possible. Some questions to consider.

Is the person living or dead?
In what field of medicine does the person work?
Does the person work at a university or research institution, or in a
    hospital?
Has the person published any books or journal articles?
In what country does the person live?

Often the only information about a person is a listing in a society roster or an address in a journal article. This is especially true for people who are just becoming established in a field.

The biographical sources and directories discussed in this chapter are examples of major sources. In addition to these sources, the librarian may refer to directories of professional societies and, the most obvious and frequently overlooked source, the telephone directory. The following sources are primarily for physicians and scientists in the United States, with a few examples of directories to scientists in Great Britain and other countries.

United States

13.1 *American Men and Women of Science*. 18th ed. New York, Cattell/Bowker, 1992/93. 8 vols.

American Men and Women of Science (AMWS) provides biographical sketches of 122,817 scientists from the United States and Canada in an alphabetical arrangement, with more than 7,000 scientists listed for the first time in this edition. The list includes 19,476 individuals in the medical sciences and 36,476 in the biological sciences. Selection for inclusion is based on (1) achievement by experience or stature derived from doctoral or current research; (2) published scientific research (or the judgment of peers for classified research); or (3) attainment of a position of substantial responsibility requiring a scientific background equivalent to the first two criteria. The directory provides brief biographical information, professional experience, present position, professional memberships, and major publications. Inclusion in the directory is by nomination and evaluation by other scientists, based on the individual's research and publications. A special feature of this directory is a necrology section at the end of each volume. Introductory information includes tables presenting geographical distribution, age, and number of scientists by discipline. Also included are the 1990 and 1991 recipients of the Nobel Prize, Crawford Prize, Charles Stark Draper Prize, National Medals of Science, and National Medals of Technology. Volume 8 includes an index by discipline and within each discipline a geographical listing of names. The printed directory of *AMWS* is in a three-year cycle. However, like many other directories its contents are available for online searching through BRS, ORBIT, and DIALOG, with frequent updating possible, and on CD-ROM as part of SciTech Reference Plus. Searching is by keyword of the discipline and subject, as well as by other elements of the biographical sketch of each scientist. Whether a library will continue to purchase the printed directory, provide access online or on CD-ROM to potentially more up-to-date information, or both, should be specified in the reference collection development policy.

13.2 *American Medical Directory*. 33d ed. Chicago, American Medical Association, 1992. 4 pts.

The 33d edition of *American Medical Directory* includes data gathered on more than 644,000 physicians through June 3, 1992, and provides information on all physicians in the United States and its possessions. American

Medical Association (AMA) members are listed in boldface type along with Doctors of Osteopathy who are AMA members. The first part of the directory is an alphabetical listing of physicians, giving their city and state of residence. The other three parts make up a geographical register by state and city that provides coded information about each physician: address, year of birth, medical school and year of degree, year of licensure, year of national board certification, specialty board(s), society membership, and type of practice. Full listings deciphering the codes are in a special section. Additional information includes officials of the AMA and AMA Auxiliary.

Purchase of the 33d and subsequent editions is available in print format 4 volumes) or on CD-ROM and requires a licensing agreement guaranteeing that information in the directory is for reference purposes only. Such restrictions may limit the availability of this directory in libraries because the directory will not be sent to libraries that refuse to either sign the licensing agreement or sign with modifications to the license. Although libraries treat the latest edition of this directory as a reference work and control its access and use, the very restrictive language of the license may prevent libraries from signing on principle, because librarians do not closely monitor "in library use" of library materials whether in print or on CD-ROM. Libraries do, however, display copyright compliance notices making clients aware of their obligations when using this directory.

13.3 *Directory of Medical Specialists*. Chicago, Marquis. Vols. 1-25, 1939-1991/92. 3 vols. Annual through 1986/87. Biennial, 1988/89- . Kept up-to-date between editions by biennial supplements.

13.4 *Official American Board of Medical Specialists (ABMS) Directory of Certified Medical Specialists*. Evanston, IL, American Board of Medical Specialists, 1986- . 7 vols. Biennial. Formerly: *ABMS Compendium of Certified Medical Specialists*.

The *Directory of Medical Specialists*, which now appears in three volumes, lists physicians certified by twenty-three recognized medical specialty boards sponsored by national societies and the corresponding scientific sections of the AMA. Each board is listed separately with a brief historical sketch, a description of the board's purpose, certification information, and the board's address. A register of members by state and city follows. A brief biographical sketch, based on information solicited by questionnaire, contains many abbreviations. In addition to information on medical school, internship, residency, and postdoctoral education, the individual's clinical training and professional memberships(s) are listed. The third volume is a name index that lists the physician's city, state, and specialty. A physician certified by more than one board will be listed for each, but biographical information will be listed only under one specialty. This directory is frequently useful when a client wants to know how "good" a physician is. It may be reassuring for a client to see which physicians are certified and to read about their education and professional training.

In seven volumes, the *American Board of Medical Specialists (ABMS) Directory of Board Certified Medical Specialists* considers itself the "only official biographical directory authorized by all 23 medical specialty boards and the American Board of Medical Specialists" (Introduction). The 1992/93 edition is updated through June 1992 and includes listings for 420,000 physicians certified by at least one of the twenty-four specialties (the American Board of Psychiatry and Neurology certifies in two specialties). Information found in this directory is similar to that found in the *Directory of Medical Specialists*; however, the information is presented in a different format. Because these publications appear biennially, many libraries have continued to subscribe to both titles. Volume 7 of the *ABMS Directory* provides an index of diplomates and a table showing the geographical distribution of diplomates. The *ABMS Directory* is available online at the American Board of Medical Specialists, where it is kept updated. That is the only location for information on diplomates who do not wish to have their names and biographies listed in the publication.

Richards and Barnes [1] highlight the history of these two publications and their relationship to the American Board of Medical Specialists. They point out the inconsistencies of the directories, which base their content on largely unedited questionnaires from individuals. Both Larkin [2] and Richards point out the more complete listing of physicians in the *ABMS Directory*. Ease of use and a lower price give further advantage to the *ABMS Directory*, however, the *Directory of Medical Specialists* remains a valuable source of information for board certified physicians, with more complete professional histories for many physicians. In 1993, these directories were combined into one directory, *Official American Board of Medical Specialists (ABMS) Directory of Certified Medical Specialists*, with the volume numbering continuing as that of the *Directory of Medical Specialists*, volume 26.

The following works are representative of directories of professional societies. Each organization has criteria for membership and lists only those individuals who have applied for or been sponsored for membership and meet the qualifications. While not the directory of a professional society, *Who's Who in Health Care* requires professional criteria for inclusion.

13.5 *Yearbook*. Chicago, American College of Surgeons, 1953- . Irregular. Kept up-to-date between editions with supplements.

13.6 American College of Healthcare Executives. *Directory: A Biographical Dictionary of the Membership*. Chicago, American College of Hospital Administrators, 1960- . Biennial. Formerly: *Directory: A Comprehensive*

Biographical Directory of the Entire Membership Including an ACHA District Index, 1960-1985.

13.7 *American Dental Directory.* Chicago, American Dental Association, 1947- . Annual.

13.8 *AVMA Directory.* Chicago, American Veterinary Medical Association, 1984- . Biennial, even-numbered years. Formerly: American Veterinary Medical Association. *Directory,* 1943-1983.

13.9 *Directory of Members.* Bethesda, MD, Federation of American Societies for Experimental Biology, 1964/65- . Annual.

13.10 *Who's Who in Health Care.* 2d ed. Rockville, MD, Aspen Systems Corporation, 1981.

The *Yearbook* of the American College of Surgeons provides brief biographical sketches of members, including hospital affiliations and titles. Some foreign physicians are listed. Members are not necessarily certified by the American Board of Surgery, but all must meet the requirements of the College to be listed as fellows. The *Yearbook* includes a section on the College's articles of incorporation, bylaws, fellowship requirements, candidate groups, past and current officers, and deceased members. Supplements published between editions include a listing of Officers, Board of Governors, and Fellows admitted since the last edition of the *Yearbook,* and Fellows deceased since the last edition.

The *Directory* of the American College of Healthcare Executives, now in its 15th edition, provides a computerized alphabetical listing of affiliates and gives complete professional biographies for more than 23,000 health care executives. Member requirements are explicit: nominees must have either a Bachelor of Arts degree with three years of hospital administration experience or a Master of Science degree and one year of experience. Nominees are accepted for membership after having passed both the oral and written examinations. Both nominees and full members are included in the directory. Much of the information is abbreviated and lists of abbreviations are provided. Information about the College's officers, awards, and special lectures are given as well. There is a geographical index.

The *American Dental Directory,* like its medical counterpart, attempts to list all dentists, not just American Dental Association members. The coded information provides a professional biography for each dentist, including information on dental education, year of graduation, and type of practice. Also included in the directory are a number of other listings: dental schools; state, national, and world dental organizations; and the number of dentists in various countries.

The *AVMA Directory* attempts to provide professional biographical sketches of all veterinarians throughout the world, not just its members. It is organized in three sections. The first section lists veterinarians alphabetically, giving name, member status, city, state, and province or country of each. A geographical section follows, arranged by state and town, Canadian province, or country. Detailed information in this second section includes spouse's name, address and coded information for school and year of graduation, professional specialty, type of employment, and employment function. A reference section completes the volume with information on the AVMA's organization and history, other veterinary and related organizations, federal and state government agencies, and veterinary colleges.

The Federation of American Societies for Experimental Biology is an association of six member societies: the American Physiological Society, the American Society of Biological Chemists, the American Society for Pharmacology and Experimental Therapeutics, the American Institute for Nutrition, the American Society for Experimental Pathology, and the American Association of Immunologists. Its *Directory of Members* provides a consolidated alphabetical listing of all members along with their addresses and phone numbers. There is also a geographical list of members, as well as organizational information—officers, committees, and constitution—for each society.

Who's Who in Health Care brings together in one source biographical information about leaders in all aspects of health care. More than 7,000 biographies are presented in an alphabetical arrangement. Inclusion in this directory, as with the others mentioned, follows certain criteria based on either one's position of responsibility or one's meritorious contribution to health care as judged by the editorial advisory board. A geographical index and a classified index (occupations, health facilities, organizations, government, private industry, etc.) complete the volume. Individuals from the United States and Canada represent the majority of the listings, although a few representatives from other countries are also present. This directory has not been updated since the second edition.

Great Britain

Information about British scientists and physicians is frequently requested. Although the following directories cover scientists in all fields, they are somewhat dated.

13.11 *Directory of British Scientists.* 3d ed. London, U.K., Binn, 1966.
13.12 *Who's Who of British Scientists 1980/81.* 3d ed. Dorking, Surrey, U.K., Simon Books, 1980.

The *Directory of British Scientists,* covering 54,000 scientists, is the British equivalent of the *American Men and Women of Science.* "Pure science" is emphasized, and entries are given in a classified arrangement by discipline, with an alphabetical name index. Biographical information includes name, address, phone number, current position, degrees obtained, and important writings. The directory also lists scientific societies, their journals and editors, and government and private research institutions.

Who's Who of British Scientists lists 10,000 men and women in biological sciences—again, in a classified arrangement by discipline.

13.13 *Medical Directory.* London, U.K., Churchill. Vol. 1- , 1845- . 2 vols. Annual.

13.14 *Medical Register.* London, U.K., General Medical Council. Vol. 1- , 1959- . 2 vols. Annual.

These two directories of British physicians are both published annually. Both also include physicians outside Great Britain and are useful for locating physicians residing in Commonwealth countries.

The *Medical Directory*, a commercial publication, lists physicians registered with the General Medical Council. The alphabetically arranged biographies include address, education, and some publications, for physicians primarily in England, Scotland, Wales, and Ireland. It includes a geographical index as well as lists of universities, colleges, medical schools, hospitals, medical governmental offices of health, government departments, coroners, medical societies, and medical periodicals. An abbreviations list and a list of deceased practitioners from the previous year precede the main directory.

The *Medical Register* is the official listing of physicians registered with the General Medical Council to practice medicine in the United Kingdom. The alphabetical listing gives a physician's name, address, registration date, and degrees, and includes foreign medical graduates certified to practice medicine in the United Kingdom. This directory is useful for locating practitioners in the Commonwealth, especially Australia and New Zealand, albeit limited to those licensed in the United Kingdom. The *Medical Register* also provides information on certification. Introductory material includes notes on the *Medical Register* for the year, notes on overseas qualified practitioners, and several tables, including one listing the current members of the General Medical Council.

Other Countries

13.15 *Canadian Medical Directory.* Don Mills, Ont., Seccombe House. Vol. 1- , 1955- . Annual.

13.16 *Guide Rosenwald Medical et Pharmaceutical.* Paris, France, Expansion Scientifique Francaise. Vol. 1- , 1884- . Annual.

These two commercially published directories provide lists of physicians both alphabetically and geographically, although their formats are otherwise different. The *Canadian Medical Directory* provides brief biographical information alphabetically for each physician (white pages) who returned a questionnaire; included are year and school of medical degree, professional memberships, position and hospital affiliation(s), address, and telephone number. Abbreviations used in this section are listed in the front of the directory. The geographical listing (blue pages) gives the physician's name and specialty under province and city. The third section (buff pages) of the directory lists universities, societies, governmental departments, and officials, as well as miscellaneous items ranging from sexually transimitted disease regulations and poison control centers to statistics on distances and areas. Official lists of Canadian physicians are published annually by the provincial licensing authorities and are available through the Provincial Colleges of Physicians and Surgeons.

In three volumes, the *Guide Rosenwald* also has a rainbow of sections listing physicians, pharmacists, hospitals, public assistance establishments, medical laboratories, and "stations hydro-climatiques" (including the curative nature of the waters) in France. This directory also contains advertising throughout.

International

Some of the people most difficult to locate are those outside of the English-speaking countries. In addition to *Guide Rosenwald*, the following directories may be of help. However, because inclusion in these directories is selective, only well-known, deceased, or older scientists are included. The directories serve well in providing brief biographical information for those individuals they cover.

13.17 *Medical Sciences International Who's Who*. 5th ed. Harlow, Essex, U.K., Longman Group, U.K., 1992. 4 vols. Formerly: *International Medical Who's Who*. Harlow, Essex, U.K., F. Hodgson, 1980-1985.

13.18 *International Who's Who in Medicine*. 1st ed. Cambridge, International Biographical Centre, 1987.

13.19 *World Who's Who in Science*. Chicago, Marquis, 1968.

Medical Sciences International Who's Who, now in its fifth edition, provides an alphabetical listing of approximately 9,000 senior medical and biomedical scientists from ninety countries who are engaged in medical research in both public and private organizations. Subject coverage includes preclinical and clinical medicine, surgery medical specialties, social and preventive medicine, psychiatry, dentistry, and pharmacy. The main listing is an alphabetically arranged biographical listing. Information has been ascertained from questionnaires provided by the individuals and includes address, educational background, professional research interests, publications, memberships, employment history, telephone number, and full address. Retired scientists and emeritus professors have been excluded. Part two, the subject listing, lists only the scientists' names.

The *International Who's Who in Medicine* provides an alphabetical listing of health professionals worldwide. Included in this first edition are "doctors in general practice, surgeons, consultants, administrators and senior teaching staff...together with nurses, dentists, pharmacologists and those concerned with public health and rehabilitation, mental health and research" (Foreword). Biographical information is from questionnaires and provides a brief professional sketch of each entrant. Entries include personal data, current position, educational degrees, appointments, memberships, selected publications, awards, hobbies, and business address.

World Who's Who in Science lists 30,000 biographical sketches of scientists from antiquity to the present and is international in scope. Entries include personal and professional information on scientific contributions and interests. The inside front and back covers provide a list of Nobel Prize winners up to 1968.

13.20 *Current Contents Address Directory. Science & Technology*. Philadelphia, PA, Institute for Scientific Information, 1984-1987. Annual. Formerly: *Current Bibliographic Directory of the Arts and Sciences*, 1978-83; *International Directory of Research and Development Scientists*, 1968-1970; *Who is Publishing in Science*, 1971-1978.

This international directory is an outgrowth of *Current Contents* for the year—previous editions contained listings from authors who had published in the previous year—providing individual author and institutional addresses. In addition, listings are included from the *Index to Science and Technology Proceedings, Index to Scientific and Technical Book Contents, Index to Scientific Reviews*, and other ISI indexing publications in science and technology. The 1987 edition lists 1.1 million unique author addresses from 180 countries. Both first and coauthor addresses are listed when given in the source publication. This is an excellent source for locating little-known scientists who have published. The author section provides the address of the first author of a paper, taken from the reprint address accompanying a journal article, as well as abbreviated citations for books and journal articles published. The organization section of the directory is an alphabetical listing, international in scope, of more than 46,000 government, academic, industrial, and other organizations. A geographical section lists the United States by state, then other countries, with the author and organization names listed below these headings. This publication ceased with the 1987 edition, but the information is available by searching the Current Contents database on tape or CD-ROM.

DIRECTORIES OF ORGANIZATIONS

Next in frequency to requests for information about people come questions about organizations. Again, addresses and telephone numbers are most often needed, although information about an organization's structure, purpose, meetings, and membership make up a great number of requests. It is important to note, even for a recent edition, how a directory obtains update information. Directories that rely on questionnaires, for example, may have dated information if a listed organization fails to respond with current information.

13.21 *Encyclopedia of Associations.* 28th ed. Detroit, MI, Gale, 1994. 5 vols. Vol. 3, loose-leaf supplement: *Encyclopedia of Associations: New Associations and Projects.*

13.22 *Research Centers Directory: A Guide to University-Related and Other Nonprofit Organizations.* 18th ed. Detroit, MI, Gale, 1994. 2 vols. Paperbound supplement: *New Research Centers.*

13.23 *Medical and Health Information Directory.* 6th ed. Karen Bachus, ed. Detroit, MI, Gale, 1992. 3 vols.

13.24 *Encyclopedia of Medical Organizations and Agencies: A Subject Guide to More Than 11,250 Associations, Foundations, Federal and State Government Agencies, Research Centers, and Medical and Allied Health Schools.* 4th ed. Detroit, MI, Gale, 1992.

13.25 *DIRLINE (Directory of Information Resources onLINE).* Bethesda, MD, National Library of Medicine.

13.26 *World Directory of Biological and Medical Sciences Libraries.* Ursula H. Poland, ed. Munchen, K.G. Saur, 1988. (IFLA Publication 42)

For an all-purpose directory of organizations in the United States, the *Encyclopedia of Associations* is excellent. Its scope is limited to national nonprofit organizations, e.g., the parent organization of the American Cancer Society is listed, but not local, state, and regional branches or affiliates. (These are listed in the volumes of *Encyclopedia of Associations: Regional, State and Local Organizations.*) The more than 15,000 entries are in a classified arrangement—science and technology, social welfare, education, etc. In addition to the address, telephone number, and chief officers of an organization, entries include membership size, purpose of the organization, meetings or conventions, and publications. The organizational name index provides listings by significant words in the name and supplements the name with a subject if the name is not clear. For example, the American Celiac Society is found in the index under

> American Celiac Society
> Celiac Society: American
> (Nutrition) American Celiac Society

The second volume provides geographical and executive indexes to the organizations, while the third volume is a supplement providing quarterly listings to new associations and projects not in the main listing. Beginning with the 18th edition, a fourth volume on international organizations and a fifth volume on research became available. A companion volume, *Encyclopedia of Associations: Association Publications*, is also available. Each volume can be purchased separately. The *Encyclopedia of Associations* is available on CD-ROM and disk or online through DIALOG, where it is updated semiannually.

The *Research Centers Directory* presents information on research organizations; however, this directory is limited to centers that are nonprofit or university sponsored and established on a permanent basis. The 18th edition lists more than 13,000 centers in the United States and Canada. Entries are arranged by subject and include size of the staff, monies spent on research, address, and purpose of the center. Two indexes, an alphabetical index by the center's name and an institutional index of sponsoring universities, complete the main volume. A loose-leaf supplement provides updated information periodically. This directory is available online through DIALOG, where it is updated semiannually.

The *Medical and Health Information Directory* brings a great deal of information together. The complete subtitle summarizes its contents.

> A guide to more than 49,000 associations, agencies, companies, institutions, research centers, hospitals, clinics, treatment centers, educational programs, publications, audiovisuals, databases, libraries, and information services in clinical medicine, basic biomedical science, and the technological and socioeconomic aspects of health care.

Now in three volumes, this directory has expanded and improved its format. Volume 1 is a directory of organizations, agencies, and institutions; it is organized into eighteen chapters with descriptive listings and a master name and keyword index. An extensive users guide at the beginning of the volume provides information on the scope, data in each entry, arrangement, index format, and source of the information in each chapter. The contents of Volume 1 are also available for licensing on magnetic tape or disk from the publisher. Volume 2 includes listings for publications, libraries, and other information services. The nine chapters are preceded by chapter scope notes and index notes and followed by a master name and keyword index to the volume. Volume 3 covers health services, including clinics, treatment centers, care programs, and counseling or diagnostic services. Following the pattern of its companion volumes, the thirty-one descriptive chapters are preceded by an introduction, chapter scope notes, and index notes, and followed by a master name and keyword Index to the volume.

This three-volume format with chapter scope notes and name and keyword indexes is a vast improvement over earlier editions of the *Medical and Health Information Directory*. The directory brings together much useful information into a single source. It is a good choice for smaller libraries because it provides a vast amount of information that could otherwise be available only with a large collection of different directories.

The DIRLINE database provides directory information for health and biomedical organizations internationally, but primarily for organizations in the United States. Organizational coverage is broad, with government agencies, information centers, professional societies, voluntary associations, support groups, academic and research institutions, and research facilities and resources included. The file is updated quarterly and had more than 14,700 records when it was last updated in May 1993 [3]. The records contain names, addresses, phone numbers, and descriptions of services, publications, and holdings.

The information in the *World Directory of Biological and Medical Sciences Libraries* was compiled from a questionnaire sent to all countries of the world as a project of the Working Group of the Biological and Medical Sciences Libraries Section of the Division of Special Libraries, International Federation of Library Associations and Institutions. Included in the directory are nonprofit libraries worldwide in the following subject areas: biological sciences, medical sciences (including allied health), dentistry, veterinary sciences, and pharmaceutical sciences. All libraries in developing countries have been included. For developed countries, the "twenty-five major resource libraries" have been listed as "selected by each country's organization of Biological and Medical Sciences Librarians..."(Foreword).

The main directory is arranged alphabetically by country and then alphabetically within country. Entries provide name, address, telephone number, librarian, subjects included in the collections, holdings for books and bound periodical volumes, interlibrary loan availability, classification used, and union list participation. There are three appendices: (1) bibliography of national and regional directories of biological and medical sciences libraries; (2) list of associations of biological and medical sciences librarians; and (3) addresses of union lists and cooperative service centers.

13.27 *Directory of International and National Medical and Related Societies.*
Compiled and edited by G. Zeitak and F. Berman. 2d ed., completely
revised. Rehovot, Israel, PBZ Informatics; Elmsford, NY, Pergamon,
1990.

13.28 *World Guide to Scientific Associations.* 5th ed. Munich and New York,
K. G. Saur, 1990.

13.29 *Yearbook of International Organizations.* 29th ed. Munich, K. G. Saur,
1992/93. 3 vols.

A worldwide directory of voluntary and professional societies dealing
with various aspects of human and animal health, the *Directory of International and National Medical and Related Societies* provides information compiled from questionnaires on approximately 4,000 societies. Arranged by
reference number, the entries include the official name in English (when
available), foreign name, mailing address, subject category, telephone, telex
and cable addresses when available, membership, society publications,
dates and location of meetings, as well as notes on whether advertising is
accepted for publications and exhibits for meetings. There are indexes by
country, name of society, and subject. A thesaurus of subject headings
precedes the subject index. The meeting and publication information are
especially useful features of this directory.

The *World Guide to Scientific Associations* is an international directory to
associations and societies representing all fields of science and the arts. The
text of the *World Guide* is arranged geographically by continent, then by
country, with an alphabetical arrangement of more than 18,000 entries. The
directory is in German and English. Each entry includes the name of the
association or society, an abbreviated name, the year of the organization's
founding, address, telephone or telex number, president's or director's
name, and number of members. A list of subjects follows the main section
of the directory. Page numbers in this list refer to the beginning of the subject
listings in the index, arranged geographically under each subject by continent, country, and then organization names; but no page numbers are given
referring back to the main directory, making the index tedious to use. The
World Guide does not include a name index by organization or a listing of
organizations alphabetically under subject. The international scope of the
World Guide is its primary strength.

The *Yearbook of International Organizations* is not limited to science and
the arts. The first volume of the current edition has an alphabetical arrangement in which there are 24,171 entries. These include 4,982 "conventional"
international organizations—essentially, an organization must have a minimum of three countries participating in its founding, aims, structure,
membership, officers, congresses, and financial backing. The organization
must also have a permanent address. There are 15,350 other organizations,

1,312 recently reported or proposed organizations, 738 religious orders, and 1,789 treaties included in the single alphabetical listing. In addition to name and address, each listing contains a description of the organization and information on publications of the organization. The alphabetical arrangement also includes abbreviations and other language titles that serve as cross-entries to the main listing. There are thirteen appendices, including a publications index that lists the publication name and reference number of the publishing organization listed in the alphabetical list. The second and third volumes, published as 10th edition 1992/93, include geographic indexes and subjects, global action networks, and a classified directory by subject and region.

The *Yearbook of International Organizations* provides more information about each of the 19,519 organizations it lists, as well as more complete and easier-to-use indexes than the *World Guide*. Both directories are useful in locating information about organizations outside the United States.

13.30 *American Hospital Association Guide to the Health Care Field.* Chicago, American Hospital Association, 1973- . Annual. Formerly: *AHA Guide to the Health Care Field,* 1972-73. Formerly: *Guide* issue of *Hospitals.*

13.31 *Canadian Hospital Directory.* Ottawa, Ont., Canadian Hospital Association. Vol. 1- , 1953- . Annual.

The *AHA Guide* is one of the most useful directories available, providing an "annual directory of hospitals, multi-hospital systems, health-related organizations and AHA members" (Cover). Major sections are color coded and include separate tables of contents at the beginning of each section. Section A (white pages) lists U.S. hospitals registered with the American Hospital Association (AHA) and osteopathic hospitals listed by the American Osteopathic Association. Arrangement is geographical by state and city, then alphabetical by hospital. Government hospitals outside the United States are also included. Each listing, in addition to the address, telephone number, and chief administrator, provides coded information on the hospital's facilities, service, governing structure, and size of staff. Accreditation by the Joint Commission on Accreditation of Hospitals (JCAH) and membership in the American Hospital Association are indicated. Brief statistical information on inpatient data (beds, admissions, census, percent occupancy), newborn data (bassinets, births), and expenses (total, payroll) are also provided. Section B (blue pages) lists AHA membership, including offices, officers, historical data, institutional members, personal members, and associate members. Section C (buff pages) lists other health organizations, agencies, and universities and schools offering educational programs in health fields. An index to all three sections and a list of abbreviations (green pages) used in the *Guide* make it a valuable reference source for hospital information. An abridged *Guide* is available on disk (3-1/2 inch or 5-1/4 inch), with optional program and table disks also available.

The *Canadian Hospital Directory* presents similar information for Canadian hospitals. Its geographical format is in eleven sections for the ten provinces (arranged west to east) plus the Yukon and Northwest Territories. Maps accompany each section, identifying towns that have hospitals. The information for each hospital is arranged geographically within each section by town or city, with the name, address, and telephone numbers for each institution, a code identifying its ownership and operating body, the licensure, and the year it was established. Brief statistics, number of beds and bassinets, personnel, and annual budget are provided to indicate level of activity. Chief administrators and department heads are also named.

Additional sections provide tables on the number of beds by type of service and group sizes, on comparison of provincial hospital plans, and other information such as outpatient health services, poison control centers, provincial hospitals and health associations, educational programs for health personnel, associations of Canadian teaching hospital members, hospital construction, and hospital associations and allied organizations. A buyers guide provides information on hospital equipment and supplies. This section also has an index to advertisers by product and service, a listing of advertisers and distributors, and a general advertising index.

EDUCATION DIRECTORIES

Frequently, information is requested about professional health schools. The professional associations formed by these schools and their administrators provide timely and accurate information about their programs, admission requirements, and curricula. Some examples follow.

13.32 *Admission Requirements of U.S. and Canadian Dental Schools.* Chicago, American Association of Dental Schools, 1964/65- . Annual.

13.33 *State Approved Schools of Nursing—R.N., Meeting Minimum Requirements Set by Law and Board Rules in the Various Jurisdictions.* 25th ed. New York, National League for Nursing, 1967- . Annual. Formerly: *State-approved Schools of Professional Nursing.*

13.34 *Medical School Admission Requirements, United States and Canada.* Washington, DC, Association of American Medical Colleges, 1951- . Annual. Formerly: *Admission Requirements of American Medical Colleges, Including Canada,* 1951-1964/65.

13.35 *AAMC Directory of American Medical Education.* Washington, DC, Association of American Medical Colleges, 1967- . Annual.

Admission Requirements of U.S. and Canadian Dental Schools lists information for the fifty-nine U.S., one Puerto Rican, and ten Canadian dental schools. Introductory chapters on "Dentistry as a Career" and "Planning a Dental Education" are followed by a geographic directory, arranged by states, territory, and provinces, as appropriate. Within the geographic arrangement, schools are listed alphabetically.

For each school, information is given on the basic program, admission requirements, selection factors, financial aid, estimated costs for four years, and admission timetable for the next incoming class. In addition, the characteristics of the most recent entering class are given, and names and addresses for further information on admission, housing, financial aid, and for some schools, minority affairs, are provided.

State Approved Schools of Nursing—R.N. is also a geographic listing. However, the information is presented in tabular form with abbreviations and codes. In all, 1,422 schools are listed for programs leading to an R.N. diploma, associate degree, or baccalaureate degree in the United States and territories. Alphabetically listed under each state are the name of the school, chairman or director of the program, address, telephone number, type of program, National League for Nursing (NLN) accreditation status, administrative control, latest enrollment, admissions, and number of graduates. Summary tables are given by state for the number of programs, admissions, and so on. A second section lists baccalaureate programs offering a major in nursing to R.N.s who have graduated from associate degree or diploma nursing programs. A directory of boards of nursing for the states and territories, as well as an alphabetical index by name of school, complete the volume. The NLN also publishes a number of other directories on nursing education and individual directories on the three R.N. programs, as well as licensed vocational nursing (LVN) and graduate programs.

Medical School Admission Requirements also presents a geographical arrangement of listings. Included are member schools of the Association of American Medical Colleges (AAMC). The information for each AAMC school in the United States, Puerto Rico, American University in Beirut, and Canada is presented in a similar format to that of the *Admission Requirements of U.S. and Canadian Dental Schools* (*see* 13.32). Brief descriptions of the curricula, entrance requirements, selection factors, financial aid, and information for minorities are followed by a timetable for application, estimated expenses for one year, and information on the most recent entering class. Ten introductory chapters discuss such topics as the New Medical College Admissions Test (New MCAT), the nature of medical education, and information for applicants not admitted to U. S. or Canadian medical schools who are still interested in pursuing a medical career abroad.

Complementing *Medical School Admission Requirements* is the *AAMC Directory of American Medical Education*. The bulk of the directory is a

geographical listing of the schools. For each school, the following information is provided: name, address, type of institution (public or private), total
enrollment, clinical facilities, university officials, medical school administrative staff, and department and division section heads. Other sections of
the *Directory* provide information on the AAMC organizational structure
and activities, Council of Deans, Council of Academic Societies, Council of
Teaching Hospitals, Organization of Student Representatives, and other
members. An index to individuals mentioned in all sections of the *Directory*
is also included.

13.36 *World Directory of Medical Schools.* 6th ed. Geneva, Switzerland,
World Health Organization, 1988.

The *World Directory* is in its sixth edition and provides information, based
on a questionnaire sent to governments and individual schools, for medical
schools in 127 countries and areas. Information on criteria for practicing
medicine in thirty-two countries without medical schools is provided.
Information is current for 1983/84. The *World Directory* is arranged by
country, providing the names and addresses of each school. Other pertinent
information includes the date instruction began, admission requirements,
length of medical studies, degrees awarded, language of instruction, and
number of students admitted and graduated in 1983. Information is presented in English and French. "Annex," an appendix, lists each country
with the page in the directory where listings begin for that country, the
number of medical schools in each country, and the country's population.
In addition to the *World Directory of Medical Schools*, the World Health
Organization publishes directories for other health schools, including veterinarians, animal health assistants, dentists, dental auxiliaries, pharmacists, and postbasic and postgraduate nursing.

13.37 *Directory of Residency Training Programs Accredited by the Accreditation Council for Graduate Medical Education.* Chicago, American Medical Association, 1978/79- . Annual. Formerly: *Directory of Accredited
Residencies.*

The *Directory of Residency Training Programs* covers much more than its
title indicates. Arranged in five major sections, it provides introductory
information on such topics as the National Resident Matching Program
(NRMP), basic information on the accreditation process, and information
for foreign medical graduates. Requirements for accreditation are outlined
in section two for forty-eight medical specialties. Section three provides
summary statistics on graduate medical education in the United States. The
fourth section, the bulk of the directory, provides a geographical listing of

accredited programs. Included in this listing are the chief of the service or program director, statistical information about that service, and the number of positions available. Five appendices complete the volume with information on combined medicine or pediatrics programs, certification requirements, medical licensure, a list of U.S. medical schools, and abbreviations used in the *Directory*.

A disk format of the directory information, AMA-FREIDA (*American Medical Association Fellowship and Residency Electronic Interactive Database Access System*), is available from the AMA. Updated annually in August, this database provides listings of residency programs certified by the AMA Medical Education Group. Information on programs varies. Those programs that are "listing in-depth institutions" provide detailed information on facilities, the educational environment, the work environment, and compensation and benefits. Information available on "non-listing" programs includes program number and name; program director's name and address (convenient for printing address labels); program start dates; summary institution information; person to contact for applications; accredited length of program; number of years offered in program; and the total number of budgeted positions. A manual is provided; however, menus guide individual access to the program.

The biographical sources and directories listed above are only a few of the vast number available. In the United States, directories of physicians, other health personnel, services, and organizations are often issued by regions, states, counties, and cities. A library should maintain directories of these local resources first, for a great number of its directory questions will undoubtedly be for local people and places. Again, the telephone directory can be an invaluable resource, and a library should maintain current telephone books for its immediate and surrounding communities.

REFERENCES

1. Richards DT, Barnes SJ. Comparative review: ABMS compendium of certified medical specialists and directory of medical specialists. Bull Med Libr Assoc 1989 Jan;77:91-5.

2. Larkin J. Book review ABMS compendium of certified medical specialists. Med Ref Serv Q 1987;6(3):99-100.

3. NLM Technical Bulletin 1993 May-June;272:2.

CHAPTER 14

History Sources

Judith A. Overmier

The cumulative nature of historical reference sources and the increase in new sources in response to growth in the study of the history of the health sciences result in an extremely well-documented field, with a reference work for almost every need. The reference tools range from general, introductory-level works to highly specific, esoteric, and sophisticated ones. The former group, which are described in this chapter, are particularly well suited to be approached first for the basic-level questions. These introductory-level questions are the kind most frequently encountered in the typical health sciences library setting. They usually can be answered with use of the local catalog and a handful of reference tools. Generally, the introductory-level tools in this field are straightforward and easy to use. They are ideal for teaching the novice patron methods of access to the history of the health sciences. Patron independence in using the tools can be achieved swiftly.

Experienced users with comprehensive research needs begin with these basic tools and progress to more sophisticated reference tools than are treated here. This group of users is no longer small in number; it is composed mainly of professional health sciences historians and their graduate students, physicians who pursue history on a professional level, and a rapidly increasing number of interdisciplinary scholars.

The more numerous patrons remain those at the introductory level; they fall into two categories: medical and nonmedical. The medical group includes students, residents, and interns, who typically make infrequent use of historical materials. Physicians also use historical materials as an adjunct to their current research and teaching.

In health sciences libraries affiliated with an academic institution, nonmedical patrons easily can become the largest part of the clientele. This group includes students in the premedical program, and undergraduates,

graduates, and faculty in other disciplines. Use by noninstitution affiliated patrons is common also, particularly with the increase in the number of independent scholars. Other users include personnel from museums or media offices and members of the lay community.

The greatest number of historical questions involve either the need for biographical information, often with portraits, or for subject-related information. This category includes requests for "all the materials on_____," "something on_____," "the most important material on_____," or "the first information on_____"—frequently accompanied by a request for an illustration of the given topic. Another large category of questions concerns older books, their care and repair, and in particular, their monetary value. Frequently, the patron will be seeking bibliographic verification or a location for a specific item. In addition, questions are asked about definitions, eponyms, and quotations.

After satisfying the basic-level patron needs, librarians may need to consult other refererence tools. Accordingly, this chapter is arranged in those groupings: biographies, portraits, bibliographies, illustrations, rare books, library catalogs, dictionaries and encyclopedias, and guides to reference tools in the history of the health sciences.

BIOGRAPHICAL SOURCES

An array of biographical tools for the history of the health sciences must provide coverage for all centuries, all geographical areas, all health sciences specialties, and all the practitioners—ordinary or famous. No single tool can accomplish this, of course, and as a result there is a myriad of biographical tools, each covering some portion of biographies.

International

14.1 Hirsch, August, ed. *Biographisches Lexikon der hervorragenden Aerzte aller Zeiten und Volker.* 2d ed. Berlin, Urban and Schwarzenberg, 1929-1935. Reprint: Munchen, Urban and Schwarzenberg, 1962. 5 vols. Supplement.

14.2 Fischer I., ed. *Biographisches Lexikon der hervorragneden Aerzte der letzten funfzig Jahare.* Berlin, Urban and Schwarzenberg, 1932-1933. Reprint: Munchen, Urban and Schwarzenberg, 1962. 2 vols.

14.3 New York Academy of Medicine Library. *Catalog of Biographies.* Boston, MA, G. K. Hall, 1960.

14.4 Wellcome Institute for the History of Medicine, London. *Subject Catalogue of the History of Medicine and Related Sciences. Biographical Section.* Munchen, Kraus International, 1980. 5 vols.

The works by Hirsch and Fischer are two of the most important biographical tools because of their international coverage of earlier centuries. Both are arranged alphabetically and include some bibliographical information. Hirsch covers to 1880, and Fischer continues the work to 1930. The *Bibliography of the History of Medicine* (*see* 14.20) also contains a biographical section with coverage that is geographically and chronologically comprehensive.

The New York Academy of Medicine's *Catalog of Biographies* is limited in scope, listing only the monographic biographical materials held by that library. It still is a useful source for pre-1954 citations. However, it and many other standard modern sources have been eclipsed by the *Biographical Section* of the Wellcome *Subject Catalogue*. This is a comprehensive index to biographies published from 1955 to 1977 in monographs, journal articles, obituaries, etc. This essential reference tool is international in scope, indexing biographies of physicians living from the earliest times to the present.

United States

Although only American tools are listed here, they are representative of tools available from other countries. A similar list could be generated for England, for instance, complete with the same problems of hiatus in coverage.

14.5 Thacher, James. *American Medical Biography.* Boston, MA, Richardson & Lord, 1828. 2 vols. in 1. Reprint: New York, DaCapo, 1967.

14.6 Williams, Stephen W. *American Medical Biography.* Greenfield, MA, L. Merriam, 1845. Reprint: New York, Milford House, 1967.

14.7 Atkinson, William B. *The Physicians and Surgeons of the United States.* Philadelphia, PA, Robson, 1878. Seconded, 1880. Philadelphia, PA, Brinton; under title: *A Biographical Dictionary of Contemporary American Physicians and Surgeons.*

14.8 Watson, Irving A. *Physicians and Surgeons of America.* Concord, NH, Republican Press Association, 1896.

14.9 Stone, R. French. *Biography of Eminent American Physicians and Surgeons.* 2d ed. Indianapolis, IN, Hollenbeck, 1898.

14.10 Kelly, Howard A., ed. *A Cyclopedia of American Medical Biography...from 1610-1910.* Philadelphia, PA, Saunders, 1912.

14.11 Kelly, Howard A. and Burrage, Walter L. *American Medical Biographies.* Baltimore, MD, Norman, Remington, 1920.

14.12 Kelly, Howard A. and Burrage, Walter L. *Dictionary of American Medical Biography.* New York, Appleton, 1928.

14.13 Holloway, Lisabeth M. *Medical Obituaries: American Physicians' Biographical Notices in Selected Medical Journals before 1907.* New York, Garland, 1981.

14.14 Kaufman, Martin; Galishoff, Stuart; and Savitt, Todd L., eds. *Dictionary of American Medical Biography.* Westport, CT, Greenwood Press, 1984. 2 vols.

Biographical tools quite frequently are limited geographically by country, state, or city. Usually, there are many tools for a geographical area, such as these selected for the United States, none of which entirely duplicate the coverage of the others.

Thacher, the earliest American compiler of biographies, was followed by a number of 19th- and early 20th-century biographers, all of whom acknowledged his influence. Both Thacher's and Williams' works contain alphabetically arranged biographies of deceased physicians. Some portraits are included.

Atkinson and Watson preferred to write about living physicians. Their works include autographs as well as portraits. Biographical entries in these books are arranged randomly, rather than alphabetically, with indexes provided.

Biography of Eminent American Physicians and Surgeons includes both living and dead physicians, along with signatures and portraits. Stone returned to the practice of alphabetical arrangement.

Just after the turn of the century, Howard Kelly instituted a series of American medical biographies, the last of which included 2,049 deceased physicians from the 17th century to 1927. It is necessary to retain all three editions due to Kelly's practice of deleting entries in later editions or of including a name entry but referring the reader to the biographical material in an earlier edition.

In spite of the number of biographical tools, gaps in coverage remain. Typically the gap is either a lacuna of time or the omission of physcans of lesser importance. Modern compilers, such as Holloway, are eliminating time gaps that have long hampered reference work in American medical biography and also are moving toward comprehensiveness by including each physician identified. *Medical Obituaries* includes brief biographical information and citations to sources of obituaries for 17,350 physicians deceased before 1907. While this seems a large increase over Kelly's 2,049, Holloway points out that it includes but a small portion of American physicians who lived prior to 1907. Kaufman's *Dictionary of American Medical Biography* covers 500 individuals deceased prior to 1976. It begins to fill other lacunae by including women and blacks; nonpracticing participants such as biochemists, medical educators, and hospital administrators; and most importantly, participants in nontraditional medicine, such as health faddists, patent medicine manufacturers, and unorthodox practitioners.

Specialties

Increasingly, biographical tools also are limited by area of specialty within the health sciences professions, such as these selected for nursing.

14.15 Bullough, Vern L.; Church, Olga Maranjean; and Stein, Alice P., eds. *American Nursing: A Biographical Dictionary*. New York, Garland, 1988.
14.16 Kaufman, Martin, et al., eds. *Dictionary of American Nursing Biography*. Westport, CT, Greenwood Press, 1988.

These are the first biographical dictionaries for nurses. Together they provide standard biographical information for 273 individuals, fewer than half of whom appear in both.

PORTRAITS

There is a high demand for portraits of historical figures. Most of the biographical works listed to this point in Chapter 14 include portraits.

14.17 New York Academy of Medicine Library. *Portrait Catalog*. Boston, MA, G.K. Hall, 1959- . 5 vols. Supplement 1, 1959-1965; supplement 2, 1966-1970; supplement 3, 1971-1975.
14.18 Wellcome Institute for the History of Medicine. *Portraits of Doctors and Scientists in the Wellcome Institute of the History of Medicine. A Catalogue* by Renate Burgess. London, Wellcome Institute for the History of Medicine, 1973.
14.19 Royal College of Physicians of London. *Portraits*. Gordon Wolstenholme, ed. London, Churchill, 1964-1977. 2 vols.

The most extensive published source of portraits is the New York Academy of Medicine's *Portrait Catalog*. It records that library's holdings of more than 14,000 original portraits, paintings, woodcuts, engravings, and photographs. Its greatest usefulness is its more than 229,000 citations to portraits in journals or monographs, both primary and secondary sources.

There are a number of other printed sources to portrait collections of institutions, such as the Wellcome Institute and the Royal College of Physicians of London. The latter includes black-and-white photographic reproductions of the library's portrait holdings, which consist chiefly of members of the Royal College.

BIBLIOGRAPHIES

Current and retrospective indexes are necessary to provide access to the secondary works in the history of the health sciences. The most important are the *Bibliography of the History of Medicine, Current Work in the History of Medicine,* and what essentially is its compilation, the *Subject Catalogue* of the Wellcome Institute.

14.20 *Bibliography of the History of Medicine.* Bethesda, MD, National Library of Medicine. No. 1- , 1965- . Annual, 5-year cumulations.

14.21 *HISTLINE (HISTory of medicine onLINE).* Bethesda, MD, National Library of Medicine, 1969- .

14.22 *Current Work in the History of Medicine.* London, Wellcome Historical Medical Library. No. 1- , 1954- .

14.23 Wellcome Institute for the History of Medicine, London. *Subject Catalogue of the History of Medicine and Related Sciences.* Munchen, Kraus International, 1980. *Subject Section,* 9 vols.; *Topographical Section,* 4 vols.

14.24 Erlen, Jonathan. *The History of the Health Care Sciences and Health Care, 1700-1980: A Selective Annotated Bibliography.* New York, Garland, 1984.

14.25 Miller, Genevieve, ed. *Bibliography of the History of Medicine in the United States and Canada, 1939-1960.* Baltimore, MD, Johns Hopkins, 1964.

14.26 Roland, Charles G., comp. *Secondary Sources in the History of Canadian Medicine: A Bibliography.* Waterloo, Ontario. Published for the Hannah Institute for the History of Medicine by Wilfrid Laurier University Press, 1984.

14.27 Chaff, Sandra L., et al., comps., eds. *Women in Medicine; A Bibliography of the Literature on Women Physicians.* Metuchen, NJ, Scarecrow Press, 1977.

The *Bibliography of the History of Medicine* is an annual publication with five-year cumulations. It covers 1964 to date. Arranged by subject, it is not as easy to use as one might wish, due to the broadness of subject terms and their modernization. Nevertheless, it is a major source because it indexes monographs, portions of monographs, composite works, and journals. It is usually consulted first in a reference search.

The National Library of Medicine's online form of the *Bibliography of the History of Medicine* is HISTLINE. The time lag for inclusion of published items into HISTLINE is considerably shorter than the printed version; thus it can be used whenever more recent materials are required. The same problems with the *Bibliography's* subject headings exist with HISTLINE, but are alleviated by the increased searching possibilities online. In addition, there are not enough subject headings assigned to each item. This subject heading problem restricts preciseness in sophisticated computer searching. As the database grows, manual searching of printed sources will become more tedious and use of HISTLINE can be expected to increase.

The *Subject Catalogue* of the Wellcome Institute is a compilation of twenty-four years of the *Current Work in the History of Medicine*. The *Subject Catalogue* is the world's most comprehensive index to secondary materials in the history of the health sciences. It is updated by the quarterly issues of *Current Work*, which in 1991, unfortunately, converted to arrangement in broad subject categories, indexing with MeSH terms. These tools provide subject, geographic, and name access to monographs and journals.

Erlen's bibliography extends coverage selectively to earlier secondary monographic materials. Arranged by MeSH descriptors and thoroughly indexed, it provides annotated coverage of more than 5,000 citations to secondary materials. It also provides subject access to dissertations and theses on the history of the health sciences.

There exist many bibliographies of secondary works that are narrower in scope than the ones listed here. Miller's *Bibliography* is an example of one limited by geographical area and by chronological period. It is invaluable as an initial source for local history. Roland's bibliography updates and expands the Canadian portion of Miller's work. Another common limitation is subject, such as *Women in Medicine*. This source is international in scope, covers the 18th century through December 1975, and provides an annotated bibliography which includes biographical and historical information.

14.28 *Index Catalogue of the Library of the Surgeon-General's Office.* Ser. 1-5. Washington, DC, U. S. Government Printing Office, 1880-1961. 61 vols.

14.29 Norman, Jeremy N., ed. *Morton's Medical Bibliography: An Annotated Checklist of Texts Illustrating the History of Medicine (Garrison-Morton).* 5th ed. Aldershot, Hants, U.K., Scolar Press, 1991.

14.30 Cordasco, Francesco. *American Medical Imprints, 1820-1910.* Totowa, NJ, Rowman & Littlefield, 1985. 2 vols.

14.31 Rutkow, Ira Michael. *The History of Surgery in the United States, Volume 1, Textbooks, Monographs and Treatises.* San Francisco, Norman Publishing, 1988.

14.32 Russell, K.F. *British Anatomy, 1525-1800: A Bibliography of Works Published in Britain, America, and on the Continent.* 2d ed. Winchester, U.K., St. Paul's Bibliographies, 1987.

14.33 Emmerson, Joan Stuart. *Translations of Medical Classics: A List.* Newcastle-upon-Tyne, U.K., University Library, 1965.

Works that identify primary as well as secondary sources are useful due to their comprehensiveness. The *Index Catalogue* is the most comprehensive of these, recording the holdings of the National Library of Medicine, the world's largest medical library. It provides such a wealth of primary materials on medical subjects that the problem becomes one of selection, rather than identification of materials. *Morton's Medical Bibliography*, undoubtedly the most heavily used reference tool in the field, provides the selection. This bibliography is arranged by subject, and it lists, with brief annotations, the first and most significant works in all aspects of every basic and health sciences field. More specialized bibliographies of primary sources are abundant. The works by Cordasco, Rutkow, and Russell are examples of sources limited by geographic, chronologic, and subject areas.

Once one has identified the classic work for a subject, it often causes consternation to find that it is published in a language other than English. Emmerson's *Translations*, although in need of updating, is a useful list of translations of these works.

ILLUSTRATIONS, AUDIOVISUAL AIDS, ARTIFACTS

Explorations of a subject area often result in a request for an illustration. There are several illustrated histories that are commonly used in answering this type of reference question.

14.34 Lyons, Albert S. and Petrucelli, R. Joseph II. *Medicine: An Illustrated History.* New York, Abrams, 1978.

14.35 Cowen, David L. and Helfand, William H. *Pharmacy: An Illustrated History.* New York, Abrams, 1990.

14.36 Ring, Malvin E. *Dentistry: An Illustrated History.* New York, Abrams, 1985.

14.37 New York Academy of Medicine Library. *Illustration Catalog.* 3d ed. Boston, MA, G.K. Hall, 1976.

Lyons and Petrucelli produced the earliest and most inclusive of these magnificent, illustrated historical surveys, followed by volumes on dentistry by Ring and on pharmacy by Cowen and Helfand. However, the New York Academy's *Illustration Catalog* provides the most extensive coverage. Arranged by subject, this catalog records holdings and provides citations to illustrations in books and journals. The third edition lists 25,048 illustrations.

Illustrations, audiovisual materials, and artifacts are frequently used for teaching and research, and reference tools are needed to guide patrons to them.

14.38 Apple, Rima D., comp. *Illustrated Catalogue of the Slide Archive of Historical Medical Photographs At Stony Brook.* Westport, CT, Greenwood Press, 1984.

14.39 Eastwood, Bruce. *Directory of Audio-Visual Sources: History of Science, Medicine, and Technology.* New York, Science History Publications, 1979.

14.40 Connor, J.T.H., comp. *The Artifacts and Technology of the Health Sciences: A Bibliographic Guide to Historical Sources.* London, Canada, University Hospital, 1987.

14.41 Davis, Audrey B. and Dreyfuss, Mark S. *The Finest Instruments Ever Made: A Bibliography of Medical, Dental, Optical and Pharmaceutical Company Trade Literature, 1700-1939.* Arlington, MA, Medical History Publishing Associates I, 1986.

Apple's catalogue indexes more than 3,000 slides by personal name, institutional name, photographer, geographic location, medical or surgical conditions, date, and subject. Eastwood's *Directory,* although out-of-date for purchasing information, can be used to identify existing audiovisual sources. It is arranged by subject and entries include an abstract of the contents as well as a physical description of the material. A useful bibliography of secondary sources about artifacts, arranged by broad subject headings, is provided by Connor. Davis and Dreyfuss focus on the trade literature, identifying and locating copies of trade catalogs, which are wonderful sources of information about artifacts and illustrations of them.

BIBLIOPHILIC TOOLS

Questions regarding historical books are common and continual. The monetary value of a given book is by far the most frequent book question encountered. Questions about the technical aspects of the physical book are also encountered fairly often.

14.42 *Bookman's Price Index.* Daniel McGrath, ed. Detroit, MI, Gale. Vol. 1- , 1964- . Annual.

14.43 *Book Auction Records.* London, Dawson. Vol. 1- , 1902- .

14.44 *American Book-Prices Current.* New York, Bancroft-Parkman. Vol. 1- , 1894/95- .

14.45 Carter, John. *ABC for Book Collectors.* 3d. ed. London, Hart-Davis, 1961.

14.46 McKerrow, Ronald B. *An Introduction to Bibliography for Literary Students.* Oxford, Clarendon Press, 1927. Reprint: 1967.

14.47 Beeson, Alain, ed. *Thornton's Medical Books, Libraries and Collectors: A Study of Bibliography and the Book Trade in Relation to the Medical Sciences.* 3d ed. Aldershot, U.K., Gower, 1990.

14.48 Horton, Carolyn. *Cleaning and Preserving Bindings and Related Materials.* 2d ed. Chicago, American Library Association, 1969.

14.49 Waters, Peter. *Procedures for Salvage of Water-Damaged Library Materials.* Washington, DC, Library of Congress, 1975.

Librarians may be able to locate a price in recent dealers' catalogs or in *Bookman's Price Index,* which compiles entries from bookdealers' catalogs. *Book Auction Records* and *American Book Prices Current,* which compile entries from auction-house sales, also may be used.

Definitions of such technical abbreviations as "t.e.g." and most other common physical terms for books may be found in *ABC for Book Collectors.* The physical makeup of the book is best described in McKerrow's publication, which is an ideal beginning source for questions regarding such things as collations, signatures, watermark placement, and irregularities in paging.

Beeson's revision of the classic *Thornton's* is an important historical resource for questions dealing with the development of the medical literature and its dissemination.

Patrons concerned about the proper care or repair of books can be served well with Horton's *Cleaning and Preserving Bindings and Related Materials.* More frequently, concern arises after a disaster has occurred. Patrons with wet and moldy books may best be helped with Waters's *Procedures* manual which gives explicit directions for drying books and treating mold.

LIBRARY CATALOGS

Catalogs of libraries are most useful for verifying bibliographical information and for locating copies of specific works. The *Index Catalogue* (*see* 14.28) is the catalog of choice for locating copies of materials, due to the comprehensiveness of the NLM collections and the library's commitment to making materials available in photocopy or microfilm, if necessary.

14.50 Wellcome Historical Medical Library. *A Catalogue of Printed Books in the Wellcome Historical Medical Library.* London, Wellcome Historical Medical Library, 1962- . 3 vols.

14.51 Durling, Richard J., comp. *A Catalogue of Sixteenth Century Printed Books in the National Library of Medicine.* Bethesda, MD, National Library of Medicine, 1967. Supplement, 1971.

14.52 Krivatsy, Peter, comp. *A Catalogue of Seventeenth Century Printed Books in the National Library of Medicine.* Bethesda, MD, National Library of Medicine, 1989.

14.53 Blake, John B., comp. *A Short Title Catalogue of Eighteenth Century Printed Books in the National Library of Medicine.* Bethesda, MD, National Library of Medicine, 1979.

14.54 New York Academy of Medicine. *Author Catalog of the Library.* Boston, MA, G.K. Hall, 1969. 43 vols. Supplement: 1974, 4 vols.

14.55 Countway Library of Medicine. *Author-Title Catalog of the Francis A. Countway Library of Medicine.* Boston, MA, G.K. Hall, 1973. 10 vols.

14.56 Osler, Sir William Bart. *Bibliotheca Osleriana: A Catalogue of Books Illustrating the History of Medicine and Science.* Oxford, U.K., Clarendon Press, 1929. Reprint: Montreal, McGill-Queen's University Press, 1969.

14.57 Eimas, Richard J., comp. *Heirs of Hippocrates.* 3d ed. Iowa City. Published for the University of Iowa Libraries by the University of Iowa Press, 1990.

14.58 Wygant, Larry J. *Truman G. Blocker, Jr. History of Medicine Collections: Books and Manuscripts.* Galveston, TX, University of Texas Medical Branch, 1986.

14.59 Hoolihan, Christopher, comp. *An Annotated Catalog of the Miner Yellow Fever Collection.* Rochester, NY, University of Rochester School of Medicine and Dentistry, Edward G. Miner Library, 1990.

Major collections, such as those at the Wellcome Institute, the New York Academy of Medicine, and the Countway, have published catalogs which are invaluable for verifying sources and locating them. The NLM catalogues of printed books from *incunabula* through the 18th century supplement the *Index Catalogue* and provide updated approaches to selected segments of NLM's extensive collection. Bibliographies of smaller collections often are equally well-known, such as the *Bibliotheca Osleriana.* Locating copies in nearby libraries is becoming increasingly important to scholars conscious of the expenses of travel, so catalogs such as *Heirs of Hippocrates,* the *Blocker History of Medicine Collections,* and *An Annotated Catalog of the Miner Yellow Fever Collection* are a significant augmentation of more comprehensive works.

DICTIONARIES AND ENCYCLOPEDIAS

Unearthing the historical roots or sources of medical terms, eponyms, quotations, etc. for patrons can be quite a challenge. Fortunately there are many reference works designed to provide an answer to this kind of question. Only a few of the most frequently used are listed here.

14.60 Strauss, Maurice B., ed. *Familiar Medical Quotations*. Boston, MA, Little, Brown, 1968.

14.61 Jablonski, Stanley. *Jablonski's Dictionary of Syndromes and Eponymic Diseases*. Malabar, FL, Krieger, 1991.

14.62 Firkin, B.G., Whitworth, J.A. *Dictionary of Medical Eponyms*. Park Ridge, NJ, Parthenon, 1987.

14.63 Magalini, Sergio I.; Magalini, Sabina C.; and de Francisci, Giovanni. *Dictionary of Medical Syndromes*. 3d ed. Philadelphia, PA, J.B. Lippincott, 1990.

14.64 Kelly, Emerson Crosby. *Encyclopedia of Medical Sources*. Baltimore, MD, Williams & Wilkins, 1948.

14.65 Skinner, Henry Alan. *The Origin of Medical Terms*. 2d ed. Baltimore, MD, Williams & Wilkins, 1961. Reprint: New York, Hafner, 1970.

14.66 Haubrich, William S. *Medical Meanings: A Glossary of Word Origins*. San Diego, CA, Harcourt Brace Jovanovich, 1984.

Familiar Medical Quotations (*see* 8.38) is patterned after general quotation books, is easy to use, and includes the common quotations usually sought. The Jablonski (*see* 8.37), Firkin, Magalini (*see* 8.35), and Kelly books (*see* 8.40) are sources for the origin of eponyms and syndromes. Each is arranged alphabetically by name and provides citations to the primary sources. The irreplaceable classic *Origin of Medical Terms* (*see* 8.9) and the more recent *Medical Meanings* (*see* 8.10) contain a few eponyms also, but mainly are concerned with the etymology of medical terms. The standard medical dictionaries are generally fairly good for providing definitions of earlier terminology.

Comprehensive introductory sources for very entry-level questions are scarce. In the past these questions were often answered from introductory textbooks, but there are no current, comprehensive textbooks and only a few appropriate reference tools are available.

14.67 McGrew, Roderick E. *Encyclopedia of Medical History*. New York, McGraw-Hill, 1985.

14.68 Walton, John; Beeson, Paul B.; and Scott, Ronald Bodley, eds. *The Oxford Companion to Medicine*. Oxford, Oxford University Press, 1986. 2 vols.

Both McGrew and Walton provide good overviews of the history of medicine, arranged alphabetically by subject.

INTERDISCIPLINARY SOURCES

14.69 Gillispie, Charles Coulston, ed. *Dictionary of Scientific Biography.* New York, Scribner's, 1970-1980. 16 vols., including Supplement and Index.

14.70 *ISIS Cumulative Bibliography: A Bibliography of the History of Science Formed from ISIS Critical Bibliographies 1-90, 1913-1965 and 91-100, 1965-1974.* London, Mansell, 1971- .

14.71 *Historical Abstracts.* Santa Barbara, CA, ABC-Clio Press.

14.72 *America: History and Life.* Santa Barbara, CA, ABC-Clio Press.

14.73 Trautmann, Joanne and Pollard, Carol. *Literature and Medicine: An Annotated Bibliography.* Rev. ed. Pittsburgh, PA, University of Pittsburgh Press, [1982].

14.74 Overmier, J.A. and Senior, J.E. *Books and Manuscripts of The Bakken: A Library and Museum of Electricity in Life.* Metuchen, NJ, Scarecrow Press, 1992.

14.75 Rodin, Alvin E. and Key, Jack D. *Medicine, Literature, and Eponyms: Encyclopedia of Medical Eponyms Derived From Literary Characters.* Malabar, FL, Krieger, 1989.

14.76 Corsi, Pietro and Weindling, Paul. *Information Sources in the History of Science and Medicine.* London, Butterworths, 1983.

The *Dictionary of Scientific Biography* is the most authoritative modern source for biographies of well-known physicians who contributed to science at large. The entries are complete, often lengthy, scholarly, and include brief bibliographies of primary and secondary sources.

The *ISIS Cumulative Bibliography* is an excellent index to the literature of the history of science, including an enormous amount of secondary source material relevant to the history of the health sciences. It is indexed by subject, with volumes on institutions and on personalities. Historical Abstracts and America: History and Life are databases that between them index secondary sources for all time periods and countries. They index much material on the history of the health sciences that does not appear in the specialized indexes of the field.

Primary sources are also increasingly interdisciplinary and locating health sciences materials in unexpected library collections is facilitated by catalogs such as the Bakken's. Its collection of electricity in life is heavy in electrical physiology, neurology, and therapeutics, for example.

Trautmann's bibliography indexes secondary sources on literature and medicine, a rapidly growing interdisciplinary research field. Rodin's encyclopedia of eponyms also reflects the growth of interest in that field.

Corsi provides a guide to information sources in science that will aid health sciences librarians in understanding the field and locating additional interdisciplinary sources.

GUIDES TO REFERENCE SOURCES

14.77 Blake, John B. and Roos, Charles A., eds. *Medical Reference Works, 1679-1966; A Selected Bibliography.* Chicago, Medical Library Association, 1967. Three supplements, 1970-1975.

14.78 Smit, Pieter. *History of the Life Sciences: An Annotated Bibliography.* New York, Hafner, 1974.

There are innumerable other reference tools in the well-documented field of history of the health sciences. Although they have been omitted in this highly selective introduction, there are, in fact, excellent reference works for foreign-language materials, for pre-18th century medicine, and for many health sciences specialities such as nursing, surgery, and pharmacy. Those reference tools are identified and described in Blake and Roos and in Smit.

READINGS

Bruce N. Searching the history of the health sciences. Med Ref Serv Q 1982 Fall;1:13-35.

Gnudi M. Building a medical history collection. Bull Med Libr Assoc 1975 Jan;63:42-46.

Zinn NW. Special collections: history of health sciences collections, oral history, archives, and manuscripts. In: Darling L, ed. Handbook of medical library practice, v. III. 4th ed. Chicago: Medical Library Association, 1988.

CHAPTER 15

Grant Sources

Pamela Broadley and Jo Anne Boorkman

In today's economy, there is an increasing opportunity for health sciences librarians to play an important role in assisting health professionals and institutions to meet their funding needs. Whether the library user is researching the availability of support for a research project, a travel grant, "bricks and mortar" funding for a major construction project, or seed money to start a new program, in order to offer effective service, the librarian must be familiar with the complex structure of the grant-making world, along with the equally complex array of information sources in this area.

There is a wide range of information sources available that deal with the different grant-making organizations. Sources vary in terms of funding sectors included, comprehensiveness, level of specificity, format, disciplines covered, and frequency of updating. The grant seeker's primary purpose is to locate appropriate funding agencies likely to be interested in a specific project. This task will involve surveying federal programs in the relevant field and, if advisable, examining the foundation and corporate arenas through a geographic or subject approach to identify likely contributors. The grant seeker will need to discern how closely the proposed project matches a foundation's or agency's interests and funding patterns.

There are three types of publications that will be useful in this process, regardless of which sector the applicant ends up approaching. These include grantsmanship guides, directories, and indexes. This chapter will concentrate on directories that encompass both government and private funding sources.

MULTISECTOR DIRECTORIES

15.1 *Annual Register of Grant Support*. 24th ed. Wilmette, IL, Register Publishing, Macmillan Directory Division, 1991. Annual.

This multidiscipline directory covers more than 3,500 support programs and fellowships of government agencies, public and private foundations, corporations, community trusts, unions, educational and professional associations, and special interest organizations. While not comprehensive, this directory contains entries for various special interest organizations, such as the American Diabetes Association, that are not found in some of the other major sources. It provides a good place to start. The directory has a classified arrangement and four indexes: subject, organization and program, geographic, and personnel. The introduction discusses types of grant-supporting organizations, and there is a chapter on program planning and proposal writing. The "Life Sciences" chapter includes medicine and other health sciences specialties.

> 15.2 *Directory of Research Grants.* 18th ed. Phoenix, AZ, Oryx Press, 1993. Annual.
> 15.3 *Directory of Biomedical and Health Care Grants, 1993.* 7th ed. Phoenix, AZ, Oryx Press, 1992.

These two sources are part of an array of grant-oriented Oryx Press products. The former is more comprehensive and includes more than 6,000 listings of research programs. Entries are arranged alphabetically with subject, sponsoring organization, and sponsoring type (e.g., nonprofit organization, foundation) indexes. The *Directory of Biomedical and Health Care Grants* lists 3,061 funding programs in the seventh edition, with the same format and indexes as *Directory of Research Grants*. Entries include information from

> (1) the sponsor's update of previously published program statements included in prior editions of GRANTS publications; (2) questionnaires sent to sponsors whose programs where not included in previous editions; (3) other materials published by the sponsor and furnished to Oryx. Updated information for U.S. government programs includes new and revised program information published in the latest edition of the *Catalog of Federal Domestic Assistance* (Introduction).

The GRANTS database from which these publications are printed is available through DIALOG and on CD-ROM from the publisher with bimonthly updates. Larger libraries that serve clientele with broad subject interests will be more interested in having the *Directory of Research Grants* available; smaller libraries with clientele strictly in the health sciences will find the *Directory of Biomedical and Health Care Grants* more appropriate because it singles out those sponsoring organizations that support the health care fields specifically.

FEDERAL FUNDING SOURCES

One caveat for grant seekers is that sources of federal funding should be explored before turning to foundations. This sequence is necessary because foundations tend to avoid duplicating federal programs and because the federal government still plays a major role in the total funding picture, in spite of well-publicized federal spending cutbacks.

The grant seeker will find some significant differences between the application process for private and federal funds. Federal agencies usually have standardized application forms, whereas foundations tend to provide the grant writer with only general application guidelines allowing more flexibility in the proposal. Furthermore, as a matter of public policy, all federal grant opportunities are announced in advance, while printed material about foundation and corporate giving may be scarce—especially for small grant-making organizations.

Because two major, comprehensive government publications on federal support exist, reference service in this area of funding could be viewed as a deceptively simple enterprise: For contract opportunities, one would consult the *Commerce Business Daily (CBD)* (Washington, DC: U. S. Government Printing Office) and for grants, the hefty *Catalog of Federal Domestic Assistance (CFDA)* (Washington, DC: U. S. Government Printing Office, 1971-). However, this approach discounts the fact that government programs are in a constant state of flux with changing funding levels, program status, and application procedures prevailing. Furthermore, a variety of materials published by individual federal grant-making agencies supplement program information in the *CFDA*. Then, too, the commercially produced sources on government funding should be consulted. Some of these publications are informative and help the grant seeker cope with the changing federal scene; others are simply duplicated government publications being sold at inflated prices. For example, Ready Reference Press is currently marketing a *Directory of Federal Aid* series. These volumes contain reproductions of *CFDA* sections, each at twice the cost of the entire government publication. The *Commerce Business Daily* has two sections that are of possible interest to health sciences clientele: A, which covers "Experimental, Developmental, Tests, and Research Work"; and Q, which covers "Medical Services." A practical option for health sciences librarians is to search *CBD* online via DIALOG when an appropriate query is made.

Effective information service in the federal funding arena begins with a basic knowledge of the agencies supporting biomedical projects. The Public

Health Service supports the bulk of biomedical investigations. The six major grant-making agencies within the Public Health Service are

1. National Institutes of Health (NIH);
2. Alcohol, Drug Abuse, and Mental Health Administration (AD-AMHA);
3. Centers for Disease Control and Prevention (CDC);
4. Health Services Administration (HSA);
5. Food and Drug Administration (FDA); and
6. Health Resources Administration (HRA).

With its mission to improve human health through research, the National Institutes of Health programs "are oriented principally toward basic and applied scientific inquiry related to the cause, diagnosis, prevention, treatment, and rehabilitation of human diseases and disabilities; the fundamental biological processes of growth, development, and aging; and the biological effects of the environment" [1]. In addition, the National Science Foundation and the Environmental Protection Agency both administer funding programs of potential interest to the health sciences professional.

15.4 National Institutes of Health. *NIH Guide for Grants and Contracts.* Washington, DC, U. S. Government Printing Office, 1966- . Annual.

15.5 *Biomedical Index to PHS-supported Research.* National Institutes of Health, Divisions of Research. Washington, DC, U. S. Government Printing Office, 1988- . Annual. Formerly: National Institutes of Health. *Research Awards Index.* Washington, DC, U. S. Government Printing Office, 1976-1987.

The *NIH Guide for Grants and Contracts* is the primary source for NIH awards. It contains relevant NIH policy information as well as new program announcements. Supplements to the *Guide* appear frequently and concentrate on contract opportunities, thus offering a welcome alternative to pursuing the *Commerce Business Daily.* Because of the often close deadlines attached to RFPs (Requests for Proposals), an even better alternative is the availability of the *Guide* online directly from NIH or through local Telenet access. GRANT LINE, as it is called, contains three main sections: (1) short news flashes that appear without any prompting; (2) bulletins that are for reading; and (3) files that are intended for downloading. The ten files are

1. General NIH information, acronyms, receipt dates.
2. Various indexes to *NIH Guide* and Requests for Applications (RFA) schedule.
3. Weekly issues of *NIH Guide* for 1990.

4. *NIH Guide*, 1991, New Electronic Format.
5. E-GUIDE, 1992, Weekly Electronic Editions.
6. NIH program announcements and guidelines.
7. Full text of 1990 RFAs available electronically.
8. Full text of 1991 RFAs available electronically.
9. Full text of 1992 RFAs available electronically.
10. NIH telephone directory, for extramural use.

The *Biomedical Index to PHS-supported Research* provides another means for determining which agency to approach with a proposal. It lists all grants and contracts awarded by the biomedical research programs throughout the Department of Health and Human Services (DHHS) from the CRISP (Computer Retrieval of Information on Scientific Projects) database. The key to the index's usefulness is the 7,000 term *Medical and Health Related Sciences Thesaurus* that permits extremely specific subject access to the award listings in which the project title, principal investigator, and funding agency can be found.

FOUNDATION FUNDING

A private foundation is a nongovernmental, nonprofit organization with funds usually coming from a single source such as an individual family or corporation. These funds are managed by the foundation's directors or trustees to "maintain or aid educational, social, charitable, religious, or other activities serving the common welfare primarily by making grants to other nonprofit organizations" [2]. In the United States, there are approximately 22,500 private foundations falling into four basic categories: independent, company sponsored, operating, and community. Briefly, independent foundations award grants from an endowment established by a single donor or family, and giving may or may not be restricted by geographic or subject area.

Company-sponsored foundations manage funds provided by a profit-making corporation and are inclined to make awards in the neighboring communities of the sponsoring company. An operating foundation usually makes few external grants; instead it uses endowment funds to conduct its own research or social welfare programs. As the name implies, community foundations are publicly supported and make grants to charitable organizations in the local community.

Unlike the federal government, which generates a constant stream of funding announcements, foundations do not usually issue lists of grants to be awarded in the upcoming months. In fact, depending on the size of the foundation, it may be difficult to locate any specifics at all about an organization's giving priorities.

Tracking down appropriate foundations is not a trivial exercise. No matter what the requirements of a particular proposal, the Foundation Center publications are the most highly recommended resources in the area of grantsmanship. Located in New York City, the Foundation Center's mission is to collect information on private foundations and then distribute this information through its publications and library collections. For referral purposes, the librarian should be aware of this organization's nationwide network of reference libraries where extensive grant information collections are maintained and open to public use. A list of these cooperating collections may be found in any of the Foundation Center reference tools. For background on seeking foundation grants, *Foundation Fundamentals: A Guide for Grantseekers*, edited by Judith B. Margolini (New York: Foundation Center, 1991), provides information on search strategies and in-depth research on prospective foundations and how to evaluate a foundation's potential interest in a project.

15.6 *Foundation Directory.* 15th ed. New York, The Foundation Center, 1993. Annual.
15.7 *Foundation Grants Index.* 21st ed. New York, The Foundation Center, 1992. Annual.

The *Foundation Directory* features nonprofit, nongovernment organizations that have private financial backing "with at least $1 million in assets or $100,000 in annual giving" (Introduction). The 15th edition is the third to be published annually and lists 846 private and community foundations reporting combined giving of $4.85 billion in 1991. This directory is especially useful for individuals seeking funds for research and education. Entries are arranged geographically by state and include the address, date of establishment, donors, trustees, and purpose of the foundation, as well as its fields of interest and financial assets. Also included is grant application information. Indexes provide access by

1. Names of persons associated with the foundations, such as donors, trustees, and administrators.
2. Geographic location.
3. Types of support, e.g., annual campaigns, building funds, conferences and seminars.
4. Subject.
5. Foundations new to the edition.
6. Foundation names.

There is a companion volume, The *Foundation Directory Part 2: A Guide to Grant Programs $50,000-$200,000* (New York: The Foundation Center,1993).

Produced from the Foundation Center's computerized file of grants of $5,000 or more awarded by about 360 major foundations, the *Foundation Grants Index* offers extremely detailed subject access by keyword, describing the many aspects of each grant. For example, through the keywords and phrases index, it is possible to identify foundations that have funded projects in pediatric neurology or alcohol abuse prevention. Foundations are listed alphabetically under the state in which they are located. Each entry contains the grant amount, recipient name and location, and grant description. Besides the highly specific subject index, there is also a recipient index that is useful to identify which foundations have funded organizations similar to that of an investigator. Since 1990, the *Foundation Grants Index Quarterly* has provided updates between editions of the *Index*. The *Foundation Directory* (updated annually), and the *Foundation Grants Index* (updated five times a year) can also be searched on DIALOG.

CORPORATE FUNDING

In addition to the independent company-sponsored foundations, corporations also distribute funds through direct-giving programs. Since 1935, the Internal Revenue Service has allowed a charitable deduction for corporate contributions up to 5% of net income. Due to the nature of direct corporate giving and the lack of published reference sources in this area, fund raising from the business sector depends heavily on personal contacts.

Given the idiosyncratic nature of corporate philanthropy and the scarcity of published information about corporate-giving policies, fund raising from the business sector is at least as challenging as tracking the small foundation grant. It is common knowledge that most corporations do not employ professionals to systematically operate the company-giving program, nor do they have well-defined philanthropic objectives or procedures for grant applications. Companies offer various reasons for this lack of definition in corporate grant programs, ranging from a reluctance to violate corporate confidentiality to the fear of a deluge of applications.

Grant seekers should be aware that even company-sponsored foundations have little autonomy and exist merely to carry out the philanthropic objectives of their sponsoring corporations. No matter how vague or nonexistent their published charitable giving guidelines, corporations tend to fund organizations serving company employees, communities in which the company operates, research in related fields, or projects that will bolster the company's public image [3]. The company's financial outlook and the special interests of the organization's principal officers also play a part in the contributions. The burden of proof is clearly on the grant seeker to demonstrate how a project is related to the company's products and services, or how the company's customers, employees, or public image could benefit from funding the proposal. The specialized directories discussed in this section are particularly suited to the corporate funding environment.

> 15.8 *Corporate Foundation Profiles*. 7th ed. Francine Jones, ed. New York, The Foundation Center, 1992.
> 15.9 *Corporate 500: The Directory of Corporate Philanthropy*. 4th ed. San Francisco, Public Management Institute, 1985.
> 15.10 *Taft Corporate Directory*. Washington, DC, Taft Corporation, 1983.

Corporate Foundation Profiles provides detailed profiles of 248 company-sponsored foundations gathered from the 1990 and 1991 *Source Book Profiles* compiled by the Foundation Center. The corporate directory provides profiles of 1,791 companies that contribute to nonprofit organizations through foundations, direct giving, or a combination of both. Part II of the directory provides information on 1,012 company-sponsored foundations that have $1 million or more in assets or annual giving of $100,000 or more based on 1989 through 1991 information. The introduction provides information on how profiles are developed and maintained on the Foundation Center's database. Subject, type of support, and geographic indexes complete the volume, which like all Foundation Center publications is quite comprehensive.

Both the *Corporate 500* and *Taft Corporate Directory* cover company-sponsored foundations and direct-giving programs. As the title implies, *Corporate 500* furnishes data on the contribution programs of the nation's 500 largest corporations. Four hundred programs, including fifty of the direct giving variety, with annual giving levels of at least $150,000, were selected for the *Taft Corporate Directory*. These directories provide comparable information on corporate-giving policies, areas of funding interest, geographic preferences, corporate financial and product information, types of activities funded, sample grants awarded, amount and range of grants, and application procedures.

The two reference tools are thoroughly indexed. However, in terms of both indexing and amount of material found in each entry, the *Taft Corporate Directory* is the most complete publication. For example, *Taft* offers more detailed information on company operating locations; analyzes the company's future giving outlook; provides a breakdown of typical recipients by subject categories such as health organization, hospitals, and medical research; and analyzes and arranges recent grants according to subject. Because corporate giving programs are often heavily tied to the personal interests of company officials, the *Taft Corporate Directory* also includes biographical information on top company officials, with indexes to these individuals by alma mater and state of birth to assist the grant seeker in developing connections with the organizations.

Although these directories are extremely useful for researching the larger corporate-giving programs, the grant researcher may wish to contact smaller corporations in the local area. For this purpose, the library user should be directed to the customary business reference tools such as *Standard and Poor's Register of Corporations* or the *Dun and Bradstreet Reference Book of Corporate Management*, both of which are available online through DIALOG.

The Taft Group provides full-text online to its newsletters, *Foundation Giving Watch* and *Corporate Giving Watch*, through NewsNet.

CANADIAN AND INTERNATIONAL SOURCES

15.11 *Canadian Directory to Foundations.* 9th ed. Norah McClintoch, ed. Toronto, The Canadian Centre for Philanthropy, 1991. Formerly: *Canadian Directory to Foundations and Granting Agencies.* 1st-6th ed., [?]-1984.

15.12 *Grants and Awards Guide/Guide de subventions et bourses.* Ottawa, Medical Research Council of Canada, 1970- . Annual.

15.13 *Reference List of Health Science Research in Canada/Repertoire de Recherches en Sante au Canada, 1991-92.* Ottawa, Medical Research Council of Canada, 1991.

15.14 Hodson, H.V., ed. *The International Foundation Directory.* 4th ed. Detroit, MI, Gale, 1986.

15.15 *International Encyclopedia of Foundations.* Joseph C. Kiger, ed. Westport, CT, Greenwood Press, 1990.

The first two publications listed are the standard Canadian sources on private and government grants. Founded in 1980, The Canadian Centre for Philanthropy is dedicated to the promotion and support of charitable activity in Canada. The organization sponsors conferences, maintains a searchable database of foundations, issues publications, and offers a host of specialized reference services to grantors and fund seekers through its associates program. As an affiliate of the Foundation Center in New York, the Canadian Centre also collects information about U. S. foundations that have supported Canadian projects. This data was incorporated into the fifth edition of the *Canadian Directory to Foundations and Granting Agencies* and has been continued in the current title. The *Canadian Directory to Foundations* contains more than 800 Canadian foundations, with information on all grants (approximately 5,800) of $2,500 or more in 1988. Indexes are arranged by subject, province and city of location, and principal foundation officers. Each entry offers the usual foundation directory categories such as grant limitations, availability of annual report, financial assets and grant range, areas of funding interest, and application procedures. Searches of the Centre's database, Foundation Search, can be requested.

The Medical Research Council, a government agency corresponding to the U. S. National Institutes of Health, is mandated to promote basic, applied, and clinical research with the aim of maintaining and improving health services. The *Grants and Awards Guide/Guide de Subventions et Bourses* documents the Council's grant-making policies and describes the various award programs with information on how to apply. Two companion publications of the Medical Research Council, *List of MRC Grants and Awards 1990/91/Liste des Subventions et Bourses du CRM 1990-91* (Ottawa, The Council, 1990), provide additional information on grants and awards.

The *Reference List of Health Sciences Research in Canada/Repertoire de Recherches en Sante au Canada* provides "information on the grants and awards made in support of health science research across Canada by federal, provincial, and voluntary agencies" (Foreword). Agencies from outside Canada, Canadian and foreign businesses, and some smaller agencies are not included. Entries include

1. List number.
2. Name of grant recipient, including co-investigators.
3. Institutional address of grantee.
4. Title of research project.
5. Funding in latest fiscal period and previous one, if applicable.
6. Effective period covered by funding.
7. Expenditure breakdown (when expenditures not normally associated with an operating grant are included).
8. Information on research trainees, their supervisor and academic degrees.
9. Names of joint sponsors.
10. Project number from granting agency.

Two indexes, one listing principal investigators and coinvestigators and the second listing the names and addresses of granting agencies listed, complete the volume.

The *International Foundation Directory* emphasizes foundations that operate internationally but also covers selected national foundations located throughout the world. Arranged by country, the directory contains 770 entries and furnishes each organization's address, brief history and description of its activities, plus limited financial data. The "Index of Main Activities" has listings for "Medicine and Health" and "Science and Technology."

The *International Encyclopedia of Foundations* includes "only the most significant foundations worldwide" outside the United States. Entries listed under the thirty-one countries included in this encyclopedia are from the foundations that were solicited for signed contributions. They provide information on the history and purpose of the foundation. Unsigned listings were prepared by the editor when sufficient information was provided by the foundation without attribution. Consequently, the amount of information on each foundation varies considerably in length and completeness. Three appendices provide a chronology, a genealogy, and a list of family-connected foundations. An index and a list of contributors complete the volume.

GRANTS TO INDIVIDUALS

One of the special situations reference librarians encounter in the area of grant information is the individual seeking funds for a personal need such as educational assistance, travel or study abroad, emergency help or medical aid, or perhaps a special research project. Largely because of stricter IRS regulations of foundation grants to individuals, only about 950 of the active foundations in this country are currently making grants to people unaffiliated with sponsoring institutions. The two sources listed below represent good starting points for the individual in search of funding.

15.16 *Foundation Grants to Individuals.* 7th ed. New York, The Foundation Center, 1991.

15.17 Williams, Lisa, ed. *Grants Register, 1993-95.* 13th ed. New York, St. Martins Press, 1992. Biennial.

Foundation Grants to Individuals contains programs arranged by grant type, including such categories as scholarships and loans, fellowships, grants for foreign individuals, general welfare and medical assistance, and grants restricted to company employees. This resource is well indexed and provides the usual descriptive information in each entry, along with lists of sample grants awarded. In addition, two informative articles appear in *Foundation Grants to Individuals*—an analysis of federal laws pertaining to this area of grantsmanship and an essay and extensive bibliography covering further sources of information on grants to individuals.

Published every two years, the *Grants Register* is broader in scope, listing information on more than 6,000 awards and grants from government agencies as well as international, national, and private organizations. Compiled for students at or above the graduate level and for others requiring further professional training, this directory includes scholarships and fellowships plus research and travel grants. While this publication emphasizes individuals in need, some of the programs make awards only through sponsoring institutions. Section six of the subject index is devoted to medical and health sciences.

REFERENCES

1. National Institutes of Health. NIH extramural programs. Washington, DC: U.S. Government Printing Office, 1980:i.

2. Introduction. In: The foundation directory. 14th ed. New York: The Foundation Center, 1992:v.

3. Kurzig CM. Foundation fundamentals. Rev. ed. New York: The Foundation Center, 1981:4.

Index